Directory of NDU Activities

Directory of NDU Activities

Compiled by Judith Lathlean with Barbara Vaughan

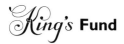

Published by
King's Fund Publishing
11–13 Cavendish Square
London W1M 0AN

© King's Fund 1997

First published 1997

ISBN 1 85717 094 6

A CIP catalogue record for this book is available from the British Library

Distributed by Grantham Book Services Limited
Isaac Newton Way
Alma Park Industrial Estate
GRANTHAM
Lincolnshire
NG31 9SD

Tel: 01476 541 080
Fax: 01476 541 061

Printed and bound in Great Britain by
Biddles Ltd, Guildford and King's Lynn

Cover photograph: *Telegraph Colour Library*
Illustrations: *Angela Martin*

Contents

Part 4: Practice-Driven Research cont.

Introduction

This directory has been compiled as a means of sharing some of the wealth of activities which have been undertaken in the Nursing, Midwifery and Health Visiting Development Units (NDUs) which have formed part of the Nursing Developments Programme at the King's Fund over the past four years. The main purpose is to bring together in one comprehensive document a picture of the range, breadth and depth of work of the units over this period of time in order that others can learn from and build on the experiences. Descriptions have been included of both small and large scale work as a means of capturing the different types of initiatives which go towards developing the service that nurses offer to patients and clients since this has been the driving force behind NDUs.

NDUs themselves have been described as pilot sites within their local context where new and innovative practices are tried and tested. Some, but not all, are at the cutting edge of practice, exploring what could be called uncharted waters such as case management, public health roles, nurse led services or clinical procedures. Others are acting as spearheads within their own organisations, exploring how well developed ideas can be applied, and often adapted for local use. In this instance the emphasis is on the implementation of national policy initiatives such as the application of clinical supervision or named nursing as well as the use of evidence based practice. The importance of recognising this continuum of activity cannot be underestimated since it is a blend of the range of work which generates the ethos of NDUs as they strive towards excellence.

Vignettes of the various activities are presented, against which readers can compare their own work as well as generating ideas for developing action plans of their own in the future. The vignettes have been grouped under headings which relate to :

Team and Staff Development – this describes those activities undertaken in order to help the team to develop as part of their endeavour to improve practice. They may be concerned with either group activities such as awaydays, team building exercises, introducing clinical supervision or individual performance review. Alternatively they may include opportunities for individual members to extend their expertise through either formal continuing education or responsibility for a specific project.

Knowledge-Based Practice – in this section examples have been included of the range of activities undertaken which relate to the use of evidence based practice and assurance of clinical effectiveness.

Developmental Work – this section, which is the largest in the directory, encompasses the project work which the teams have undertaken, often in response to a specific patient or client need or a desire to improve practice. Examples include exploring new roles, increasing the involvement of users, quality initiatives and clinical developments. Some of this development work may well form the basis of more rigorous research in the future.

Formal Research – while some units have concentrated on development work and internal evaluation others have chosen to undertake more formal research spanning a longer time period and drawing on the expertise of an experienced researcher. It is these latter activities which have been included within this section.

Dissemination and Marketing – since one of the characteristics of NDUs is that they share their work with others we have included a final section describing some of the activities which have been undertaken to this end.

Wherever possible references of published material have been included in order that readers can gain access to more detailed information. Similarly a note has been made of internal reports and papers which have been produced for local use, many of which are available directly from the Units concerned. However it must also be pointed out that both NDUs and the teams who work within them are dynamic in nature, and as time has moved on and service contracts have changed, so have some of the units, the nature of their work and the staff. Many of the people who have been involved with this programme from the outset have progressed in their careers, leaving behind a legacy of development as well as using the skills they have developed in other settings, which it can be suggested is a hidden value of NDUs. Hence new units are emerging all the time while others may shift the emphasis of their work to reflect the rapid changes which are occurring throughout the health service. Current contacts can still be found through, among other sources, the Practice Development and Research Network at the King's Fund, newly formed regional data bases and the New Roles Data Base at the University of Sheffield (SCHARR).

It would not be possible within one document to include all the work of every unit since so much has been achieved that a tome would be needed. Furthermore many of the activities are common to the units, crossing boundaries of clinical speciality and setting. Hence in some instances we have used a sample of examples from the units which demonstrate the issues related to a series of key themes. In other instances, where the work has focused on an activity which is specific to one NDU, we have included a more comprehensive coverage.

It is not intended that this directory is read from cover to cover but 'dipped into' as a means of raising ideas about development work as well as giving insight into the enormous range of activity which is being undertaken by nurses who are committed to improving the service they offer to patients and clients. Our thanks must go to all those who have contributed to this endeavour, not only for their hard work but also for their willingness to share both their successes and areas where they have experienced difficulty with others.

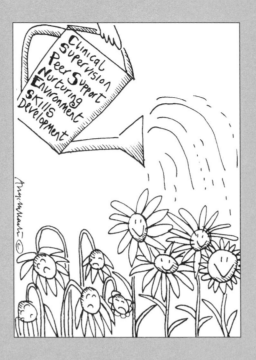

Part 1

TEAM AND STAFF DEVELOPMENT

One of the most critical features of Nursing Midwifery and Health Visiting Development Units (NDUs) is the commitment they have to giving all members of the team an equal opportunity to contribute to the development work, recognising that no one can work successfully in isolation and that everyone has a part to play. Simple though this may sound it is something which requires active management to ensure that mechanisms are established for everyone's view to be heard, for the part which each team member will play to be made explicit, for learning needs to be identified and for learning opportunities to be made available.

This first section summarises the various ways in which NDUs have addressed the vital issue of development for the team. Experience of working with the NDUs suggests that investment in team members is not a luxury but a necessity for the provision of high quality care.

In times of pressure it is an easy option to miss out time for reflection, debate or learning. Yet it can be argued that the cost of such an omission is one which cannot be afforded in the longer term. The following extract has been taken from one nurse's experience of working in an NDU rather than a more traditional ward setting. It goes some way to expressing how staff respond to the ethos of learning, enquiry and support which is so common to NDUs:

The development of something better is for me what the NDU is all about. It is far from an abstract concept – it is living and breathing in all the hearts, minds and behaviour of the staff on the unit and is passed on to all who come into contact with them. The strengths shown by leaders within the unit are those of vision, to recognise potential and to support, release and nurture that potential in a way that benefits nursing, nurses and ultimately the people we care for. Nursing is about people; our NDU is concerned with development of people as people – that is both clients and nurses.

Primary Nurse – Seaford (wards V and W) NDU 1994

Many ways have been found of helping people to enhance their knowledge and skills through both formal and informal routes. There is an expectation that time spent in development is critical to the longer term quality of care and is a legitimate part of work. Hence colleagues have supported one another and respected the value of shared and individual learning opportunities. While it would be unrealistic to suggest that these efforts have been easy to sustain there is no doubt that the impact on practice is significant, as is the resultant increase in staff satisfaction and morale. As another nurse, contrasting her experience of working in the NDU with her previous work, has said:

....At times it can be hard work and time can be short, but then progress does not come easily. Yet I have only found enthusiasm and encouragement and an attitude that is open and reflective. I am able to set my own objectives and negotiate my personal development plan, and in a wider sense I have more of a vision of where I see myself going. I had none of this five months ago

Named Nurse – Cartmel Nursing Development Unit 1994

This section has been divided into parts which relate to team development, subsuming amongst other things team building activities and organisational changes, and personal development where new skills have been learned and systems such as clinical supervision and personal development plans have been introduced. It offers a range of options which will act as a focal point for others who wish to introduce staff development strategies within their own units.

Team Development

The development of the team in NDUs has been achieved in a number of ways; for example by looking at the whole philosophy of the unit, and the part that teams and individuals should play within this; by reviewing the way in which the unit works as well as by team-building activities and engaging in team approaches to staff development. Respect for others, sharing, and effective communication have been vital within the NDU teams who have been very aware of the importance of forward planning as a joint endeavour.

Team building related to philosophy and values

For many NDUs, team development centres around the philosophy and values underpinning the work of the unit. Different aspects and avenues have been explored as a means of achieving this as shown in the following examples.

Values clarification

A focus of activity at Chelsea and Westminster Intensive Care Unit (ICU) NDU has been the clarification of values of individuals as well as the team, using an unusual 'cascade' process. The agreed purpose of developing a philosophy for this unit has been:

- to encourage nurses to share intuitive feelings and question their own value systems
- to form the basis for policies and practice and a reference to resolve conflicts and ambiguity of objectives
- to act as a first step towards the establishment of measurable standards

The main premise has been that the appropriate starting point in the development of a philosophy is that of establishing *values* which can then be translated into *objectives* and *action*. For example, for the value statement 'families, relatives and significant others are important people to patients', the specific objective is 'to involve relatives in care to the extent that they and the patient wish participation' and the action, that 'all relatives are asked about their expectations of care'.

The process involved the use of a questionnaire to all nurses to provide a baseline of knowledge. This was followed by the identification of common ground and collective values and beliefs through a cascade method and group techniques involving nurses and other members of the multi-disciplinary team (described in detail in Warfield and Manley, 1990). Small buzz groups (of four) brainstormed ideas in response to a simple values clarification exercise which included such statements as:

> 'I believe the purpose of the ITU is ...
> I believe my purpose in the ITU is ....
> I believe critically ill patients need ...
> If I was a patient in ITU I would like ...
> I believe the ITU environment for patients/staff should be...
> I believe individuals learn best when ...'

This activity has been fundamental to the development of the NDU and critical, not only in enhancing team cohesiveness but in identifying areas for future work. (Warfield and Manley 1990)

Developing the ward philosophy through group interviews

Another approach has been that of developing the ward philosophy through focus groups. The John Radcliffe Hospital NDU felt that an earlier attempt to develop a philosophy should be revisited; team members had changed and further developments had taken place since the original statement was formulated. The team was committed to involving every member in this process but recognised the difficulty of getting everyone together at the same time. As an alternative they used a series of focus groups, each meeting for about an hour, where discussions relating to the philosophy were held. In this way all team members could attend in small groups so that everyone had the opportunity to participate. All discussions were taped, transcribed and analysed. A new statement was created which was then validated by the whole team. Three broad issues were raised:

- What does the philosophy do? The team saw the philosophy as giving them a sense of shared belief which complemented their personal beliefs and guided their practice

- What are its features? The most critical feature of the philosophy was seen as its relevance to the needs of patients, highlighting the importance of using jargon free language. As a result, terms such as 'unconditional warm regard' and 'informed choice' were simplified
- What concepts are inherent in the philosophy? Five key concepts were identified including continuity, caring, partnership, choice and relations with other disciplines. Common understandings of each of these concepts emerged. Owing to their commitment to patient involvement the team has also developed a pictorial version of the philosophy which they use to introduce patients to the ward. (see Garbett 1994, 1994a)

Reflective Practice Action Group

West Dorset NDU chose the mechanism of a Reflective Practice Action Group. Their aim was to explore the organisation of care delivery – primary nursing – and roles and relationships within the unit. A local university offered to help set up the research to take place over one year. All team members were given information and the choice of taking part. The programme entailed fortnightly meetings, each with a particular theme which was explored and reflected upon. It was anticipated that this would support team development, identify aspects of nursing practice for discussion, and clarify internal and external roles and relationships. (see Graham 1995)

Peer supervision

The route adopted by Annex NDU was that of peer supervision. They viewed supervision as a way of maintaining and ensuring a high standard of care, of learning from someone more clinically experienced, and as a tool for self development. Individual supervision involved both internal and external supervisors and was based on a psychodynamic model. This supervision took place on a weekly basis, and the team has concluded that internal supervision works best in this setting in terms of the benefits to patients, team members and the team as a whole. The clinical leader had external supervision from a non-medical psychotherapist with experience of working with people who have anorexia.

Supervision needs changed during the life of the project and as team members developed. Peer supervision involved using all team members, including the clinical leader, as equals to discuss individual casework with particular reference to personal difficulties and issues which might arise for team members in their work with patients. As team members became more experienced, the need for this kind of supervision decreased, to the extent that it is now held on an *ad hoc* basis, according to need. (see Halek 1996)

Organisational changes to work as an NDU

Some of the units have looked at their whole organisation in respect of team development, with the additional motive, on occasion, of enhancing recruitment and retention of staff.

Team working

In Dewsbury NDU there has been an emphasis on developing appropriate teams of nurses in a non-traditional way. Six self-selecting members of the NDU team undertook training to develop skills as team leaders, using a modified version of the trust's *Leading and Developing your Team* package. Three teams (referred to as 'development teams') were formed and each member of the unit was invited to complete a self-perception inventory which was used, in conjunction with team-leader consultation, to build the most effective teams possible in terms of abilities and skills. The development teams were charged with the task of acting as a peer support group for the NDU nurses and with developing practice in the unit.

This approach to team leadership challenged many norms and traditions as the leaders were not all senior nurses or holders of vast clinical experience, but had received training for the leadership role. This innovative approach to team building has ensured that the skills and expertise of all members are maximised. A peer support mechanism has been introduced as well as the challenge and opportunity for developing nursing practice. (see Dewsbury NDU Annual Report 1995)

Inter-team projects

Chelsea and Westminster NDU aims to facilitate unit cohesiveness by the use of project groups which concentrate on key areas of responsibility and have membership from all the teams. They recognised a potential for reduced cohesiveness among the whole team with the introduction of primary nursing and small groups and felt the need to find ways of ensuring See also page 138 cross-team interchange.

Six such groups have been established (off-duty planning team; quality assurance co-ordinators; journal review group; marketing group (see section 5);

finance group and teaching co-ordinators' group). As an example of a project team, the teaching co-ordinators' group consists of a member of staff from each of the primary nursing teams. The purpose is to organise, co-ordinate and monitor all educational and staff development activities and meetings. This is done mainly by:

See also page 16

- encouraging staff to complete a 'teaching requirement form' to identify training needs
- organisation of a written monthly teaching rota by each teaching co-ordinator in turn.

Achievements to date include the development of a learning directory and a two-week competency based programme for D-grade staff; a shift in lunch-break patterns to ensure maximum attendance at teaching sessions; a standard of a minimum of two teaching sessions per week; development of regular individual performance reviews. (see Chelsea and Westminster Intensive Care and NDU Annual Report 1994–5)

Readjustment to team and workload

The stimulus which has driven Strelley NDU (Health Visiting) has been a recognition of previously ignored health needs of a population living in a deprived area in Nottingham, as well as difficulties with recruitment. There was also a desire to explore new models of working, with an emphasis on the contribution health visitors could make through exploring the public health role. Unlike many of the other NDUs the team at Strelley was made up of a peer group of health visitors with no line management within the team itself. Hence establishing ways in which leadership of the development and project work could be undertaken was critical.

The first step was to recruit staff and then, through extensive team negotiation within the NDU, the group agreed to redistribute and reorganise the workload to free time for one colleague to undertake public health work. The team also agreed that another team member would be responsible for managing the development work (rather than the team), acting as the main point of communication for NDU work. The unit worked with an external facilitator who initiated the development of reflective practice skills as a means of highlighting both strengths and weaknesses in their practice. Group review was incorporated in this process which has particular relevance for community staff who work in potential isolation and recognise the critical importance of peer support. A publication of case studies reported by the health visitors demonstrates how this process can be used in day-to-day practice to explore the invisible aspects of health visiting. (Boyd *et al.* 1993, Periton and Perkins 1995)

Reviewing clinical grading

The Maudsley NDU has reviewed its clinical grading in order to generate an internal clinical career structure. This was part of a system for retaining team members who were committed to developing practice which provided them with a clear structure for their own individual development. The existing establishment was examined over a six-month period, aimed at incorporating an in-house development and promotional structure. D grade primary nurses joining the unit were offered a training package to enable them to develop wider roles and skills. They could then apply for promotion to E and F grades within the following 12–18 months. Three newly created F-grade, clinical charge-nurse posts were advertised on the unit to existing staff. Needless to say this work had to be undertaken within the existing budget of the ward and required a review of the whole staffing pattern. (see Maudsley NDU Bridging Therapy: Annual Report 1993–4)

Team building activities

The importance of team building has clearly been recognised, and units have used a variety of strategies. These tend to be one of two kinds: either the use of workshops and awaydays, or by external consultancy.

Team building events

The tensions and pressures experienced by East Berkshire NDU in the early days have largely been alleviated by an emphasis on team building. This has taken the form of residential three-day workshops for F and G grade nurses with the clinical leader as a facilitator. In addition, days have been set aside for team work and weekly seminars involving many different professions. Invited guests have been helpful in promoting knowledge and cohesion.

Team building awaydays have occurred throughout the life-span of the project and continue to thrive, providing opportunities for discussions of roles and skills within the team, and reorganisation of working practices with clients and carers. Team meetings continue on a weekly basis with team members taking the lead on a rota basis. (see East Berkshire NDU Annual Report 1994–5)

Similarly, though in a very different practice setting, team building has been an essential element in Anston NDU at Rampton. This has stemmed from the special needs of the psychopathic patient group cared for on the unit who, as part of their condition, can skilfully capitalise on poor communication or relations of staff members. The unit team went through a number of staff changes during their first year as an NDU, but recognised the importance of ownership and vision in continuing their developments. It was in the second year that they convened a team-building workshop, off-site, to facilitate the process of reforming, redirecting and re-energising the team. This exercise, during which plans were set for the future and action plans devised, was a vital process in improving staff morale and renewed enthusiasm for the work. Since team involvement is central to their work the workshop has been followed by both formal team-building sessions and informal interactions where all members are asked to contribute new ideas for the future. (see Anston NDU Report 1993–4)

Weston Park (Sheffield) NDU sees team-building weekends as a vehicle to enable staff members to join together in an out-of-work setting. The relaxed atmosphere, social inter-action and physical activity enables greater understanding by individuals of the strengths and weaknesses of fellow staff members. This in turn leads to a more cohesive team on return to the workplace. The weekends are also a time when improving care and innovative change can be discussed, and appraisal of proposals that have already been implemented undertaken.

The team at Weston Park have found these weekends so valuable that they plan to continue in the future when external funding has ceased.(see Weston Park Hospital NDU Brochure)

Team building with external consultants

Annex NDU has placed a lot of emphasis on team building and team development involving the use of external consultants and facilitators. The team was started from scratch and recruited especially for the project. Along with workshop days and sessions to look at values clarification, strategic development, team roles and problem-solving, the team has also held a regular fortnightly group session throughout the work of the project, facilitated by a group analyst. This work is currently being written up to describe the life of the team, the problems it has been working with and the effect on the team of their clinical work. The report will be available in late 1997.

Team approach to staff development

Several of the units have an all-encompassing programme of professional development, with emphasis on the creation of a learning environment and wide-ranging learning opportunities. Others have concentrated on development activities in relation to a specific aspect of the unit's work. Workshops have proved a popular strategy for facilitating staff development.

A multi-faceted approach to professional development

Bowthorpe NDU illustrates a multi-faceted approach which includes:

Awaydays for primary nurses and the Clinical Leader along with a Link Tutor
Awaydays and team building for primary nursing teams
Development workshops for primary nursing teams on subjects such as customer care, communication and interpersonal skills
Personal development plans (pending in accordance with trust policy)
Continued support for formal continual education of all grades of staff, for degrees, DPNS, NVQ, ENB courses. (see Chadwick et al. 1996)

Similarly, Liverpool NDU believes that the development programme for staff must be supported by the whole team. A wide range of opportunities exists for professional development apart from the more formal courses including activities such as job exchange schemes, job rotation, in-service training, guided reading, role development and project work. (see Swift 1995)

A planned educational programme has been used by Dewsbury NDU to increase team members' knowledge in relation to the needs of the unit. For example a deficit in knowledge about paediatric care was identified. Initially one team member was given time out to undertake RSCN training and there is now a rolling programme to train the others. A wide range of other skills has been gained by team members through educational activities including the diploma in care for people with asthma, teaching and assessing courses, management of violence and aggression, drug and solvent abuse awareness and the ENB Accident and Emergency course. In addition post-graduate studies have been undertaken with a view to preparing people for practitioner lecturer posts within the department. (see Dewsbury NDU Annual Report 1994)

Creating a learning environment

Creating a learning environment for the staff has been an important aim of Glenfield NDU, based on the belief that by improving the knowledge and skills of the nurses the standard of care which they offer to patients will also be better. This links closely with the self-care philosophy which the unit follows, coupled to a nursing responsibility to ensure that patients have every opportunity to learn about their illnesses and treatments and to prepare for discharge. To this end the unit has a number of initiatives including induction programmes for new staff, a resource room, clinical supervision, ward-based workbooks, quizzes and games, teaching packages and opportunity for time out to study. (see The Glenfield NDU – the past three years, 1992–1995)

Learning opportunities

One of the key objectives for Anston NDU has been the provision of learning opportunities for team members. A questionnaire was circulated to all team members as a means of identifying their existing knowledge and skills of relevance to clients' needs. Simultaneously, information was sought about areas where it would be beneficial to develop new skills. Following this exercise links were made with the Staff Education Centre with a view to developing appropriate teaching packages as well as drawing on other sources of help. The team have developed their knowledge and skills in specific problem areas for the client group they work with such as eating disorders, self-injurious behaviour and other disruptive behaviour. Educational programmes in these and other areas such as stress management, relaxation, debriefing and assertiveness have all combined to increase the team's knowledge and confidence in undertaking their work. (see Anston Ward NDU, Rampton Hospital 1993–4)

Development of primary nursing programme

Some units have taken a key focus for their work and set up a programme of staff development to support this. For example, Glenfield NDU has established a Primary Nurse Development Programme, designed to last over a six-month period which includes four study days and five clinical supervision days with the practice development nurse. The aims of the programme are:

- to facilitate the primary nurses to understand and apply personal accountability to their practice

- to provide the primary nurses with the necessary skill and knowledge/motivation to contribute actively to create a learning environment for staff/patients
- to facilitate the primary nurse's acquisition of the necessary skills and confidence to actively involve patients in all communication processes (bedside handover, evaluation of care)
- to provide the primary nurses with the necessary knowledge and skills to reflect and learn from their practice

Evaluation of this programme has formed part of the research activity for the unit. (see Furlong 1994, 1996)

Workshops

Workshops are a common way of achieving staff development. For example Andover NDU has had a series of workshops to help and support staff to cope with the changes in the unit. These have been facilitated by experts and have covered such areas as: HIV/AIDS, breast care, aromatherapy, diabetes, stoma care, psychiatric care, bedside handover and primary nursing. The unit has also developed its on-site library resources to support the staff development. (Andover Annual Report 1994)

Similarly West Dorset NDU, in actively promoting nursing as a therapy in its own right, has held activities, workshops and discussion groups around: aromatherapy, massage and touch and therapeutic touch. As well as exploring these issues in relation to nursing, the workshops, some of which have been led by experts in these particular fields, have given the team a sense of purpose. They have also been a source of fun and stress relief. Following on from the team work, one of the primary nurses has developed her own project on massage and touch. The development of local resource people in this way is not an uncommon outcome of workshop activities and can be seen in many other units. (White 1995).

Team communication

Communication within units is vital in order to sustain team working. Traditional approaches are commonplace to the NDUs as well as the use of some more unusual approaches such as making use of technology and seeking external advice and links.

Ward meetings

Weston Park team hold regular weekly ward meetings which they see as an essential activity. While this may seem fairly basic, the team know these can be difficult to implement and sustain but they have learned that such meetings are essential for both the smooth running of the ward and to maintain some control over the way in which their work develops. (see Weston Park Hospital NDU brochure)

Recording meetings

In the Maudsley NDU, videos have been used to ensure team meetings were shared by all team members. The videos can be reviewed by members who were not able to attend or used to refresh the memory of those who were present. (see Maudsley NDU Bridging Therapy Annual Report 1993–4)

Many other units have either used tape-recordings or kept written records of all their meetings for similar purposes. The emphasis has been a commitment to ensure that all members of the team have access to information and are able to contribute their own views; a central feature of NDUs is their aim of ensuring team involvement and commitment.

External advice and links

Within Stepney NDU, advice and facilitation is available from a link lecturer from the College of Nursing. As well as being a resource for students, this provides support for the staff by improving the learning environment and enables the joint identification of learning needs within the team.

Similarly, Ashington NDU has made links with a colleague from the University of Northumbria who was seconded for a period of three months to assist in the evaluation of some aspects of the unit's work. Many units, including V and W wards, at Seacroft Hospital in Sheffield, paediatric outpatients at Southampton and the intensive care unit at the Royal Sussex Hospital in Brighton, have forged links with local universities which have proved fruitful in bringing together the skills of practice, research and education.

Links have also been made with local pressure groups and national interest groups as well as with other people who have an interest in the work of the NDU such as community health council members and local commissioners, all of whom can offer valuable advice in helping to plan development work.

Future development work

The units have used many different processes to identify development work which they will focus on in the future. The approaches are often multi-faceted ensuring that a range of different perspectives and views are taken into consideration when planning a strategy for development which will take current and future needs into account.

Identification of key project work

Within Royal Bournemouth Hospital NDU, as a result of a survey carried out with midwifery staff, four target projects were identified. These included:

- *evaluation of the team concept* – This work entailed the formal evaluation of care through a team approach using a range of tools to elicit factors including the number of contacts with the team, contacts outside the team, delivery by the team and perception of care.
- *transitional care* – Occasionally there was a need to transfer women to the neighbouring obstetric unit during labour if risk factors developed. Earlier evaluation indicated that there was room for improvement here and a working group has been exploring different means of improving transitional care.
- *midwifery input into high risk care* – This group has been seeking to identify ways of increasing midwifery input for women who are considered high risk by, for example, regular contact, drop-in centres, leaflets and so forth.
- *the SHO training package* – The importance of providing an opportunity for newly-qualified doctors to learn about normal pregnancy and childbirth has been highlighted and a midwifery-led programme introduced which will be formally evaluated, with subsequent publications.

Each working party will be responsible for planning projects in terms of time scale, objectives and evaluation criteria and will give written reports on progress. All the midwives in the unit have had the opportunity to sign up, to take part in the projects in which they are most interested. (see Royal Bournemouth Hospital NDU Maternity Unit Report 1996, Thomas 1994)

Personal Development

Another key element found in units relates to the development of individuals. This may be through a variety of individual staff development and training activities, by processes such as clinical supervision and appraisal, and Individual Performance Review (IPR) as well as through schemes which allow for individual time out for development purposes.

Staff development and skills training

The starting point for some units has been the identification of needs for development by profiling or undertaking an educational analysis. This is a precursor to the often quite extensive array of staff development activities which may include specific skills training or activities focusing on personal growth. Reflective practice seminars are just one example of the different approaches that are used.

Staff profiles

All members of staff on the Seacroft (wards V & W) NDU are provided with a staff profile when they join the unit. These profiles, with guidelines and information on how to use them, were put together by the nurses themselves and the team are actively encouraged to use them as a means of facilitating reflection. Within the profiles are IPR 'documents' and the staff, together with their supervisors, set themselves aims and objectives on a more formal basis. (see wards V and W, Seacroft Hospital NDU Second Annual Report 1994)

Educational analysis

Maximising opportunities for education and staff development has been a high priority for the Newcastle NDU. To undertake the educational analysis, staff have developed a structure using the English National Board's Higher Award framework in order to identify the skill mix and learning needs of the team related to both personal development and the clinical needs of the unit.

This has enabled the NDU to be pro-active in planning to minimise duplication and to ensure that both individual and unit needs are met. (see Royal Victoria Infirmary Annual Review 1993–1994)

Staff development

See also page 6

Chelsea and Westminster ICU NDU encourages continuing professional development by, for example, supporting involvement in external post-registration and post-graduate programmes (e.g. Diploma of Nursing, Master's and PhD); by internal provision (e.g. an induction programme for new staff and two-week competency-based programmes for D-grade staff); through staff being responsible for reviewing and critiquing key journals. Activities are organised and needs assessed through participation in all inter-team projects. In this way knowledge and skills are developed and through specific personal action plans staff are empowered. (see Chelsea and Westminster Intensive Care and NDU Annual Report 1994–5)

Cartmel NDU has produced a booklet (one of six) about their staff development activities. This is based on the philosophy that 'by promoting better and continued training and education of nurses, by looking at ways to conduct and use research to underline and legitimate practice, and by overcoming cultural barriers it is hoped the nurses in the NDU can develop themselves to realise their potential and give patients the care they are entitled to' (Gadd *et al.* 1995a). Several general initiatives foster or encourage staff development, notably: clinical supervision, information technology, client-led quality initiatives, research-based care plans, and networking. Three further pursuits are aimed specifically at staff development – staff appraisal and personal development planning; team nursing and 'key working'; and support staff to facilitate professional development. The booklet (in common with all six booklets produced by Cartmel NDU) concludes by giving a list of do's and don'ts that the unit have concluded from their experiences:

- do establish contracts for study leave and make benefits to clients clear
- do ensure a system for staff appraisal and personal development is established
- do undertake training needs analysis on an annual basis
- do raise awareness and ownership through workshops, discussion, awaydays, exchanges

- do be creative with budget to employ replacement staff or part-time facilitator
- do network ... learn from others instead of trying to re-invent the wheel
- don't be too ambitious and over-critical (Gadd *et al.* 1995a)

Skills training

Specific skills training for staff related to their work is a feature of many of the NDUs. For example, Sheffield Occupational Health NDU has supported members of the nursing staff attending an RSA counselling skills course through local colleges, as well as one and two day seminars. Other team members have attended a variety of other learning activities including stress management and aromatherapy courses. (Sheffield City Council, Occupational Health Division NDU Annual Report 1993–4)

The Michael Flanagan NDU has engaged in focused training and skill development for team members related to personal interests and to unit needs such as personal and social health education, family therapy and hypnotherapy. (Dodd and Sheehan 1994)

Byron Ward NDU has developed skills in physical assessment in order to ensure patient safety in the nursing-led in-patient unit (Evans and Griffiths 1994) and the team in Worthing NDU has developed skills in administering many cytotoxic drugs as well as in the management of lymphoedema in order to widen the service which they can offer to patients.

In these, and many other examples, the drive to develop new skills has come from the nurses themselves as a means of being able to offer a service which is more responsive to the needs of the patients or clients with whom they work.

Complementary therapy training

In Ashington (Ward 5) NDU one member of the unit has been funded to attend an aromatherapy diploma course. In addition, all staff were introduced to the concept of therapeutic massage through participation in a seven-week evening class held at a local sports centre entitled Massage for Health. By the end of two years 15 staff had attended the course.

The results of an evaluation survey indicated that the majority felt they benefited from the course, it was enjoyable, relaxing and taught them basic skills. However, lack of time to make use of these new skills in practice remains a concern. The comments made raise many questions about the problems of establishing such therapies in acute areas. Nevertheless, it has been concluded that there is potential for staff to use massage in their work by incorporating it into other elements of care. (see Ashington Annual Report 1993–94)

Reflective practice seminars

Liverpool NDU has been conducting fortnightly seminars during which nurses have presented stories of instances where they feel they have made a difference for a patient or relative. Initially, staff needed help to remember

See also page 121

positive situations but subsequently the seminars have proved to be a means of generating information about aspects of nursing practice which have often remained hidden, as well as providing an approach to staff development. This has increased self-awareness, knowledge, critical thinking and presentation skills. The seminars have been a part of a research study aimed at exploring the value of clinical nursing practice. (see Waterworth 1995a)

Clinical supervision

Not surprisingly, systems of clinical supervision are a common feature of NDUs and this has been the subject of a publication (Kohner 1994), produced as part of a series of five booklets which stem from work accomplished by the NDUs. The following entries show a range of ways in which schemes operate and also the benefits that are felt to accrue from the process. Reflective practice is central to many of the approaches as is a commitment not only to improve care but also to provide support for team members.

Guided reflective practice has been used as a form of clinical supervision in Chelsea and Westminster ICU NDU. This was developed initially by a pilot group of the team leaders, Clinical Nurse Specialist (CNS) and an external expert adviser, but has now cascaded through the team. Participation is voluntary. At the initial meeting of supervisor and supervisee, ground rules are agreed clarifying confidentiality, anonymity and honesty. The supervisee keeps a written diary related to clinical practice, using Johns (1994) *Model of Structured Reflection*. At subsequent meetings the model is used by the supervisor to guide questioning of the supervisee. The supervisor keeps notes of the ensuing dialogue, and these, along with the diary entries, provide a basis for further meetings. Future goals include the development of group clinical supervision in the unit and clinical supervision on a wider basis. To this end, the unit's CNS is facilitating two pilot groups of nurses and individuals to develop guided reflective practice within the trust. (Chelsea and Westminster Intensive Care and NDU Annual Report 1994–5, Manley 1994)

One of the main objectives for Cartmel NDU was to develop a system of clinical supervision which could be piloted on the Unit but later used throughout the trust. They separate managerial and clinical supervision very clearly and have produced a register of supervisors so that participants can select those who have the requisite skills to help them develop their practice. They do however also arrange regular meetings between the manager, clinical supervisor and supervisee to ensure there are common aims and no conflict of interest. (Gadd 1995b)

Additional developments have been:

- the introduction of recording sheets
- presentation of the work at a national conference
- training for two members of staff on an intensive two-day event, facilitated by external consultants
- negotiations with the Royal College of Nursing to develop the work into an RCN update (see Gadd & Mahood 1995)

Stepney NDU arranges for each team member to have clinical supervision every four to eight weeks which includes setting of goals and personal development planning. Closely linked with this is their reflective practice project and reflective practice writing framework, designed by a link lecturer from the College of Nursing, for use by practitioners. The project explores and develops different methods of reflection within primary health-care settings and facilitates the dissemination and continuing development of these strategies within their community health services. Introductory and follow-up workshops on the theory and skills of reflection have been successful in informing and motivating the team, community nurses and managers. Reflection is now built into the unit's evaluation strategy and is being used and further developed in many aspects of the unit's work. (Stepney Nursing Development Unit Annual Report 1994)

Clinical supervision was introduced in the John Radcliffe Hospital NDU to 'empower patients through the empowerment of nurses'. The scheme follows the King's Fund guidelines (Kohner 1994); it was established to reflect the notion of stewardship (accountability without control or compliance) and is based on reflection (Northcott 1996). The supervision structure was predominantly a cascade, with the clinical leader meeting each team leader every eight weeks, and they in turn meeting team members to provide support and encouragement, challenge and vision. No formal records were held but individuals were encouraged to keep their own notes and a number elected to generate simple learning contracts which were kept within their personal professional profile.

In the West Dorset NDU, one of the off-shoots of developing primary nursing has been the recognition of the need for reflection and support for primary nurses' practice. The primary nurses themselves felt strongly the need for time to discuss their work. The changing role of the clinical leader necessitated a different way of spending time with the primary nurses and helping them reflect accurately on their practice. Allowing time for this through clinical supervision appeared to enhance the professional approach that primary nursing advocates for nursing. Following national guidelines, the unit has developed a model with a strong reflective and developmental process. This has not been an easy development: whilst nurses themselves want clinical supervision they are only just beginning to feel confident enough to provide it for others. There are nurses on the unit who have so far decided not to receive clinical supervision, but those using it are positive about its benefits and are committed to its continued development. This work has been aided by a colleague from the local university who had undertaken similar work with Seacroft (wards V and W) NDU in the past (see below).

Supervision has been firmly established on the Seacroft (wards V & W) NDU for some time. Each nurse has a named supervisor, and the set standard is that every member of staff will have a minimum of six and maximum of 12 sessions over a 12-month period. Supervision for individuals usually occurs every four to six weeks, with hourly sessions. The supervisee shares the responsibility of organising the sessions with the supervisor. Ward W team informally evaluated what the nursing staff actually wanted from clinical supervision using a questionnaire. It is hoped that this will later be established at a more formal level, perhaps with an existing evaluation tool. This process has also been linked with the development of reflective skills (see previous entry). (wards V and W Second Annual Report 1994) (see Graham 1995)

A combined system of unit supervision, using an external facilitator, and individual clinical supervision with a minimum of monthly meetings has proved effective in the Maudsley NDU. In the former, the team has been able to discuss feelings of loss, anger and fear as well as their positive learning experiences. (Maudsley NDU *Bridging Therapy* Annual Report 1993–4)

In response to the document *A Vision for the Future* the clinical leader of East Berkshire NDU organised a three-day workshop on supervision for trust staff. Three team members were among eight who attended the first two days on individual supervision and the follow-up day which introduced group supervision. Positive outcomes have been increased use of clinical and managerial supervision throughout the trust, and development of peer supervision. During 1995 a member of the NDU was seconded on a part-time basis to the trust's training department to further develop work on clinical supervision. (East Berkshire NHS Trust 1996)

Appraisal and individual performance review

Appraisal and performance review are also part of personal development in many of the units and some examples are given below.

Self-appraisal and CANDU

Stepney NDU has developed a self-appraisal form (referred to as Stepney CANDU) to target and evaluate the dissemination of NDU information within the neighbourhood team and to identify specific training needs and help all team members contribute to achieving the aims of the NDU. Staff were asked to answer yes or no to statements which include:

- I could explain my own job or area of professional practice to other colleagues in the team or students and visitors to the team
- I could speak at a conference about my job or area of professional practice
- I could do a joint presentation or workshop (or one on my own) about the NDU; or I could do a development programme within my own team or to another group of community nurses or to other groups

Self-identified learning needs are then followed up by training and development seminars both in-house and externally facilitated and organised. (see James 1993)

Individual performance review and personal development plans as the focus of development processes

From the outset Byron Ward NDU used a system of individual performance review linked to personal development plans for all team members. Through this system each team member focused personal development on an issue which would also be of value to the rest of the unit. Dedicated time was allowed for this activity which was more commonly linked to a personal action plan than to a formal course or training. (Herbert and Evans 1991) As the unit has developed the nurse-led in-patient service the IPR system has taken on many of the features of clinical supervision. In this instance, however, there is a firm commitment to the belief that these two processes – IPR and clinical supervision – should be closely linked to ensure there is no conflict of interest between managerial and professional accountability.

Worthing NDU has developed an innovative approach to IPR using SWOT – an analysis of strengths, weaknesses, opportunities and threats. In this way, each member of staff has time to examine formally what they think are their own strengths and weaknesses, what opportunities are available to them and what may threaten their progress. This is done away from the ward and provides the opportunity for the clinical leader to give praise and offer advice regarding courses and other activities that may be available for further development. At each review, a plan is made and a date set for further review. (Day Ward, Worthing Annual Report 1994)

Ashington (Ward 5) NDU has a system which aims to help qualified nurses realise their potential to develop and contribute to a high quality service for patients. The process is a cyclical model based on an annual cycle of initial review and target setting, intermediate review, and major performance review. Each team member has at least two performance review meetings per year with his or her manager, and has a personal development plan. The IPR system was fairly well-established for qualified nurses on the unit by the second year of the programme. Towards the end of the year, staff were surveyed to find out what they thought of the system. All nine individuals said it was either of some use or was very useful to their personal and professional development. One made the following typical comment: 'I was able to see progress made and to identify and discuss areas which need improvement and new ideas. I feel that professional development is being monitored in order to achieve optimum performance'.

The benefits included the opportunity to: 'talk to someone about your workload'; 'know that you can identify your weaknesses and try to improve them'; 'know that someone is there to help you with any problems and that everything discussed is confidential'; 'confirm progress made and goals still to be met'; 'express the way you feel'; and 'explore within yourself'. In addition the system was felt to be 'morale boosting' and made individuals realise their capabilities. Nevertheless, the drawbacks included: 'the time the manager has to devote to interviews'; 'soul searching' and 'finding the right study days to improve performance'.

The trust has since introduced its own performance review and development model which is linked to performance-related pay. It is somewhat different from the NDU model and consequently some modifications are necessary to equalise the two. (see Ashington Annual Report 1993–94).

Personal time out

Allowing personal space has been important for the development of individuals within the units. At a time when resources are scarce this has not always been easy since clinical demands are high. Yet many of the teams have recognised that if they are to develop their practice then time to prepare is a necessity rather than a luxury.

Dedicated time for study and personal development

In Worthing NDU, each member of staff has half-day study per month allocated to them. This is usually taken as one day bi-monthly because of the difficulty of taking half a day each month. This time is for personal study but is also used to concentrate on project work for the NDU. (Day Ward Worthing 1994) Similarly, Stepney NDU provides the opportunity for each team member to have reflective time bi-monthly in order for them to develop ideas and action plans which will be of benefit to the unit. Some staff have used this time very actively to prepare proposals for small grants to undertake further development work, one example of which was the funding secured to explore the needs of Asian women weaning their children. (Stepney NDU Annual Report 1994) In Homeward NDU at Brighton the time out has led to a series of local 'experts' who are used as a resource by colleagues in areas such as wound management, a strategy which has been adopted by many of the other units. (Phelan *et al.* 1992)

Clinical fellowship schemes

Liverpool NDU introduced a scheme of clinical fellowships. The NDU spanned three wards and one nurse from each area became a clinical fellow for a period of six months, being freed for one day each week to contribute to a major project on the development of core-care protocols. Each fellow focused on a specific aspect of care such as nutritional needs, communication, or pain, and gained skills in undertaking literature searches, preparing the protocols under the guidance of the development worker and helping to introduce them to colleagues, thereby also gaining skills in the management of change. This was an excellent way of gaining commitment from team members over time as well as enhancing their individual skills and providing the opportunity for a large number of people to contribute to the developmental work of the NDU. (Royal Liverpool and Broadgreen University Trust NDU Final Report 1995)

Similarly, in Michael Flanagan NDU, the creation of a clinical fellows scheme has allowed a member of the team formal reduction in his clinical commitment over a full year, in order to study a specific aspect of care. The scheme is competitive with any team member able to apply. The team suggests that this openness has not only directed support and understanding of the responsibilities of the clinical fellow but has also led to a perceived value in the exploration of clinical practice. (Dodd 1994, Vaughan and Edwards 1995)

SUMMARY

The value of activities which focus on team development should never be underestimated. For example, without a shared understanding of the rights of patients or clients and their relationship with health-care workers, confusion and potential conflict can arise in day-to-day practice over shared information, flexibility of practices, access to case-notes and many other aspects of work. In the same way, as the saying goes, time to learn may seem expensive, but the cost of not knowing can be even greater. With the drive to increase the use of evidence-based practice throughout the health service it can be argued that a prerequisite is the personal development of health-care personnel. As they extend the range and breadth of their personal knowledge this will, in turn, ensure that the care offered to patients and clients is knowledge-based and of a high quality. Thus the development of staff can be seen as a means to an end. It is the underlying process through which the quality of care is enhanced.

The benefits of a systematic and planned approach to staff development do not end here. A less tangible but equally important aspect relates to the impact this can have on both staff morale and career paths. For example, one NDU has reported that the throughput of staff was slightly higher than the rest of the hospital. However when the career paths of these people were examined the majority of moves had been either for promotion or for full-time study (Northcott 1995). Similarly, reports from many NDUs indicate that, even though the pressure of work is high, they value the opportunity they have for personal development and growth which is often a reason for attracting new team members to the units.

In this section a range of different approaches has been collated in order to give an idea of the variety of work which the NDUs have undertaken. All of the units have been committed to development opportunities of one kind or another and it has been necessary to be selective since inclusion of all the work that has been done would be too lengthy. Nevertheless, the examples offered here may help other teams who wish to undertake similar activities and suggest ways in which both personal and team development can be enhanced.

References & related reading

Anston Ward NDU, Rampton Hospital *Annual Report* 1993–4

Ashington Ward 5 NDU, Second Annual Report 1993–4 Northumberland, Wansbeck District General Hospital

Chadwick D, Smith L, Simmons T, Parent A, Monks S (1996) *Building An Effective Team* Bowthorpe NDU, Norfolk and Norwich Healthcare NHS Trust

Chelsea and Westminster Intensive Care and NDU *Annual Report* July 1993–June 1994

Chelsea and Westminster Intensive Care and NDU *Annual Report* July 1994–June 1995

Dewsbury NDU *Annual Report* 1995

Dodd T and Sheehan A (1994) 'Professional Development Opportunities'. *The Briefer* Stafford, The Foundation NHS Trust

Dodd T (1994) 'A year in clinical fellowship'. *Nursing Developments News* (December) issue 9 p12 London, King's Fund

East Berkshire NDU *Annual Report* October 1994–September 1995

East Berkshire NHS Trust Behavioural Support Team (1996) *Developing Best Practice*

Evans A, Griffiths P (1994) *The Development of a Nursing-led In-patient Service* London, King's Fund

Foundation NHS Trust (1994) *Nursing in Focus – The Value of Mental Health Nursing: a strategic perspective on Clinical Nursing practice in the Foundation NHS Trust* Stafford

Furlong S (1994) 'Primary Nursing: a new philosophy' *British Journal of Nursing* 3(13) 668–671

Furlong S (1996) 'Practitioners' perceptions of primary nursing' *Professional Nurse* 11(5) 309–11

Gadd D, Colgan L, McFadden K, Collins C, Hadcroft D (1995a) *Staff Development: Participating in Change* Cartmel NDU, Mental Health Services of Salford NHS Trust (also available on Internet – front sheet Cartmel NDU)

Gadd D, Mahood N (1995b) *Clinical Supervision: a time for professional development* Cartmel NDU, Mental Health Services of Salford NHS Trust (also available on Internet – front sheet Cartmel NDU)

Garbett R (1994) 'Changing philosophy through group interviews' *Nursing Standard* 8(22) 37–40

Garbett R (1994a) 'The Focus Group interview: a flexible tool in nursing development' *Nursing Developments News* (7) London, King's Fund

Glenfield NDU *The past three years 1992–1995* (1996) Leicester, Glenfield Hospital

Graham I (1995) 'Reflective Practice: using the action learning group mechanism' *Nurse Education Today* 15(1) 28–32

Halek C (1996) 'Clinical Supervision – can you afford to be without it?' *unpublished*, Annex NDU, Pathfinder Trust

Herbert R, Evans A (1991) 'Staff appraisal and development' *Senior Nurse* 11(60) 9–11

James J (1993) *Stepney CANDU form* Stepney NDU

Johns C (1994) 'Nuances of Reflection' *Journal of Clinical Nursing* 3(2) 1–13

Kohner N (1995) *Clinical Supervision in Practice* London, King's Fund

Manley K (1994) 'Clinical Supervision: why surgical nurses need it' editorial *Surgical Nurse* (February)

Maudsley NDU 'Bridging Therapy' *Annual Report* December 1993–November 1994

Northcott N (1996) 'The significance of culture in an NDU' *Nursing Developments News* 15 3–5 London, King's Fund

Northcott N (1995) 'Career Trajectories for nurses working in NDU' Internal Report 7E NDU, Oxford Radcliffe Hospital

Periton C, Perkins E (1995) *Working in Partnership: Health Visiting in an Area of Deprivation* Strelley NDU, Nottingham Community Health NHS Trust

Phelan P, Hawkey B, Sheppard B (1992) 'Wound Management: Research Alongside Care' in Black G *Nursing Developments Work in Progress* London, King's Fund

Royal Bournemouth Hospital NDU *Maternity Unit Report* (1996) Bournemouth

Royal Liverpool and Broadgreen University Trust NDU *Final Report* (1995) Liverpool

Royal Victoria Infirmary NDU *Annual Review* 1993–4 Newcastle

Seacroft (Wards V and W) Hospital NDU (1994) *Second Annual Report*

Sheehan A (1994) 'Extending the Role of Mental Health Nurses' *Nursing Standard* 8(44) 31–34

Sheffield City Council, Occupational Health Division NDU *Annual Report* 1993–4 Sheffield

Stepney Nursing Development Unit *Annual Report* (1994)

Swift F (1995) *A Team Approach to Staff Development* Liverpool, Royal Liverpool and Broadgreen University Trust

Thomas M (1994) *Normal Delivery for Obstetric House Officers* Bournemouth, Royal Bournemouth Hospital Maternity Unit

Vaughan B, Edwards M (1995) *Interface Between Research and Practice* London, King's Fund

Warfield, Manley K (1990) 'Developing a new philosophy in the NDU' *Nursing Standard* 9(23) 24–26

Waterworth S (1995) 'Exploring the value of clinical nursing practice; the practitioner's perspective' *Journal of Advanced Nursing* 22(1) 13–17

Weston Park Hospital (1995) *NDU Brochure* p 6, Ward 3 Weston Park Hospital, Sheffield

White D (1995) *Therapeutic Touch: Caring in Practice* internal report, West Dorset NDU

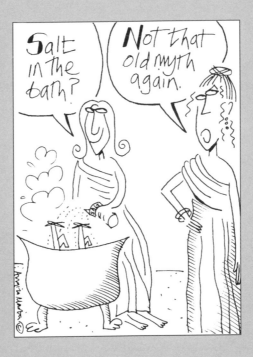

Part 2

KNOWLEDGE-BASED PRACTICE

Gone are the days when any professional practitioner could hide behind the mantle of professional mysticism denying information about recommended treatments to the passive recipient of care. With the increase in acknowledgement of patients' and clients' rights to receive care based on evidence, as well as having a voice to choose options, it is imperative that all health-care workers seek to meet these obligations. Actions must be taken through personal development which will enhance knowledge-based competency. Such changes have been welcomed by NDUs who are driven as much by patients' rights to care founded on current research as to a commitment to offer services which are effective and efficient. This is the subject of a publication on the experience of working with a range of units which summarises the different approaches taken to tackle the difference between research and practice (Vaughan and Edwards 1995).

Use of knowledge in practice is a complex process since the sources of knowledge and people's acceptance of what is legitimate are diverse. Acceptability is a critical feature from the perspective of both service users and service providers and, however effective treatment regimes may be, their value must be questioned if they are not acceptable to patients or clients. It is clear that professional practitioners in all walks of life should be able to offer people a clear purpose in their services and to outline the thinking on which they base their actions. Respect for the autonomy of recipients of care also means that services are offered in a non-judgmental way and if people wish to explore other options or refuse recommended treatments then these wishes must be respected. Such features are ones which are fundamental to the philosophy which drives NDUs.

There are some areas of care where the evidence on which practice is based is less clear cut than others and there are many areas which still require rigorous investigation. Thus there are times when care is based on a combination of both formal evidence and skilled professional judgement. Such situations can give rise to what have been called 'creative options' and it is important that such actions are captured since they may one day be subject to scrutiny through research. Actions of this kind are another feature of NDUs as they 'spot the gaps' and often, through the use of clinical supervision and reflection on action, raise the right questions about areas of practice which might later be evaluated more formally.

Having stressed the importance of basing practice on evidence it must be acknowledged that no one can be the font of all wisdom. Finding ways in which we can effectively draw on shared expertise within the context of multi-professional teams is essential in practical terms. Hence the use of agreed standards, protocols, guidelines and local experts which may have been developed at either local or national levels; these can all play an important part in day-to-day practice and are approaches which many units have taken. Making use of the information arising from centres whose main purpose is to undertake analysis of research such as the Cochrane Library (Dickson and Callum 1996) and the Centre for Review and Dissemination at York, which holds a database of abstracts of reviews of effectiveness is just one way in which expertise can be shared and time saved while responding to the challenge of ensuring that care is knowledge based.

Standards and Protocols

Developing a range of protocols is part of the standard setting and quality assurance strategy of many of the units. Sometimes more unusual approaches are used such as a method of cascading information from a specialist through the team as a means of sharing expertise. Monitoring and evaluating the standards is normally built into the process as a way of auditing care and assessing quality. The examples given below are representative of a very wide range of activity in this area which is common practice in NDUs.

Protocol development and standard setting

See also page 6

In the Chelsea and Westminster ICU NDU, protocols identify specific structure, process and outcomes standards with a research or evidence-based rationale. The protocols are used to provide a basis for clinical practice, as an educational tool and a means of standard setting and quality assurance. They are also used to feed into care-plans, thus reducing the amount of writing required. Staff have either worked individually or in groups, often on topics of special interest (e.g. endotracheal suction). Initial drafts are critiqued by the multi-disciplinary team and after a few months in use, auditing of outcome standards is attempted. The unit believes that the formulation of protocols has enabled staff to develop their research-based knowledge. This facilitates the integration of theory and practice, it results in the standardisation of practice functions, provides clear guidelines and a good educational tool to help in the provision of complex areas of care such as the management of a patient in acute renal failure requiring haemodiafiltration. (Chelsea and Westminster Intensive Care and NDU Annual Report 1994-5)

A commitment to ensuring that patients receive high quality, knowledge-based care led the Royal Liverpool NDU to a programme which focused on the development of 'core protocols for care' based on the literature available. They did however recognise that there were some areas of practice about which there is little evidence, such as using abdominal massage to ease constipation. They have incorporated a section in the protocols to record 'creative actions' in order to ensure that those aspects of clinical care which are so often ignored are captured, with the possibility of becoming a focus of research in the future. The unit devised a scheme of clinical fellows where team members from each of the wards involved participated in developing and implementing the protocols. These core protocols not only guide practice but are also used to help staff identify gaps in their own knowledge and have led to specific educational programmes being developed. It is felt that the protocols can also be used to identify areas of good practice which can then be used as bench marks for others. (see Waterworth and Byrne 1995, Royal Liverpool and Broadgreen University Trust NDU 1995)

See also page 23

Seacroft (wards V & W) NDU has produced standards for care which are used to guide care and are subject to periodic review. Two such standards relate to continence management and management of care for patients at meal times. In the latter, there is one main standard statement which is that 'every patient who dines on V Ward will receive care which enhances his/her sense of individuality within an environment that is unhurried and promotes independence'. The way in which this is fulfilled is divided into a set of criteria statements about structure (the structure of the dining area and the availability of resources); process (e.g. 'all patients will be encouraged to exercise their right to choice and this will be respected') and outcomes (e.g. 'all nurses will be responsible for the care of their allocated patients and be aware of their fluid and diet intake'). (Littlewood and Saeidi 1994)

Bowthorpe NDU has audited seven of the 12 core nursing standards using questionnaires which were piloted on the unit. These were: admission and transfer procedures, explanation of treatment, assisted bathing, induction period, analgesia (administration and effect), assessment of skin. In the process, patients' opinions were sought and their knowledge gained. As a result assessment procedures have been incorporated into care plans, and the questionnaires have been modified. (Bowthorpe NDU Annual Report 1995) Similarly Homeward NDU in Brighton has developed standards which are used to both guide and audit care. (Homeward Rehabilitation Unit 1991)

Standard setting using a cascade approach

The Royal College of Nursing's standard setting training workshops (Dynamic Standard Setting System or DYSSY) have been attended by four team members of the Stepney NDU and they have cascaded the insights and knowledge gained to the rest of the team. Both multi-professional practice-based teams and specialist groups such as health visitors and district nurses have contributed to or set appropriate standards and been involved in reviews and audits. Where 'specialists' have been involved it has been easier (in terms of time, resources and knowledge) and more effective. For example, the leader of the Well Leg Project (a district nurse) has been able to set leg ulcer care standards; a health visitor specialist in housing and homelessness has advised on a housing standard. In this way best use can be made of the specialist and thus reduce the amount of time and resources required to undertake this kind of standard setting work. (Stepney NDU Annual Report 1994)

Use of standards as a precursor to audit

The Newcastle NDU has developed a document entitled *Standards for Orthopaedic Nursing*, initially as a nursing-led initiative using the Dynamic Standard Setting System, but now as a multi-professional clinical audit tool. All standards have audit tools to monitor and measure compliance to pre-agreed criteria within a multi-professional framework and the lead which nurses have taken in this area has been of value to many others. (Laxade and Carney 1992).

Audit

*Closely allied to standard setting and monitoring is the process of audit.
The use of audit is extensive in the NDUs covering wide-ranging aspects
of work and, as the following examples demonstrate, using a variety of
different approaches within the same general principles.*

Nursing audit using Senior Monitor

Bowthorpe NDU has used the audit tool Senior Monitor (Goldstone *et al.*
1986) as they felt it addressed the areas of care which are more likely to
occur with the elderly patients who are nursed on the ward. Over a four-year
period their Monitor score moved from 73% for nursing care to a score of
83%. While it is difficult to attribute this progress to one specific change
members feel that their move to primary nursing had an important part to
play. This favourable comparison gave them a clear indication of the
progress which has been made. In response to the findings of the second
audit the unit designed and introduced new documentation in order to
improve on their recording of the evaluation of care and these records are
now used widely throughout the trust. (Bowthorpe NDU Annual Report
1994)

Audit and development

Dewsbury NDU chose to use Accident and Emergency Monitor (Dutton,
Grylls and Goldstone 1991) to audit the overall nursing care provided in the
unit. From the audit data topics were identified for which clinical standards
could be developed. This work was partly triggered by the introduction of a
standard for patients with fractured neck of femur and this led to a big
reduction in the waiting time in A and E prior to transfer to the ward.
More recent standards using DYSSY (Kitson 1990) relate to patients with
cervical or thoracic spinal injury, those with chest pain, carers of children
following sudden death and potential asthma suffers.

Internal audits

West Dorset NDU has undertaken internal audits on pain, wound management and bedside handovers. One outcome from this work was the development of a pain assessment tool which is now being used widely in the hospital (Allen 1992). Lack of time, pressure of workload and financial constraints have made audits difficult at times. However, the unit has been in discussion with the trust's audit department to utilise their skills and further work in this area is planned. (Allen 1992).

Research-based Practice

Research-based practice in the units encompasses a range of different aspects such as the development of care plans which are underpinned by research; the development of research skills through discussion of the literature and planned time out to undertake project work; provision of research-based information for patients and clients and the use of reflection to bring to light both strengths and weaknesses in care and potential deficits in knowledge. As access to knowledge is more readily available through centrally-funded initiatives such as the work of the Cochrane Collaboration in undertaking meta-analysis of research, as well as a greater emphasis being rightly placed on public accountability for care, this is an essential aspect of the work of the NDUs.

Research-based care plans

The project in Cartmel NDU was designed as a way of promoting the use of research-based practice to plan care for highly dependant clients, most of whom had been in hospital for twenty years or more. The process adopted has been:

- an annual global assessment by key workers and co-workers to review all clients' needs
- a review of the client's needs by a multi-disciplinary team six monthly
- a care planning meeting with the care team three monthly
- a critical analysis of the care plan monthly

Evaluation has been by baseline, random and yearly audit of care plans, and interviews with key workers. The outcomes so far have included: focus on choice and empowerment in clients' care plans; increase in key worker accountability; clients' care plans contain rationale for the priority-need identified and the nursing interventions; new assessment tools have been developed; extensive literature reviews have been undertaken by key workers and monthly research awareness sessions have been introduced. In an area where there is limited evidence of effective practice the team have devised a way of being able to link the actions they have instigated to the outcomes for patients in order to increase their understanding of the care process. (Gadd *et al.* 1995b)

Development of research skills through discussion of the literature and networking

In many of the NDUs, for example in Stepney, research skills and knowledge are enhanced by joint discussion of papers and research findings at project and team meetings and circulation of articles and other reading material. Similarly, Chelsea and Westminster has established a journal club where team members agree to bring articles from a range of journals to the attention of colleagues and the Cartmel team have stimulated some discussions through the Internet. (Gadd 1995)

Formal reading and reflection time

Reflective strategies such as exploring critical incidents, reflective writing and using vignettes to describe practice are commonly employed by many of the units. For example in the early days of development Truth Ward NDU helped the team to develop reflective skills through a series of workshops which were externally facilitated. (Truth Ward Annual Report 93–94) Similarly, the unit in Liverpool has used reflective processes with continuing research to explore the therapeutic nature of nursing (Waterworth 1995). In Strelley the team spent time at the outset of the project developing reflective skills with the support of a colleague from the local university as a means of clarifying their understanding of current practice and exploring ideas for development. (Boyd *et al.* 1993)

In Stepney NDU there is reading and reflection time of up to one day a month away from the practice setting. As a result many of the team have prepared applications which have been successfully submitted for funding for further project work. They see this as an essential element of their work and a means of enhancing developments and quality of care. (Stepney Annual Report 1994)

Research-based resource files

Bowthorpe NDU, like many others, has a considerable number of resource files on wide-ranging topics. As part of their overall strategy to help the team gain research skills staff read nursing journals and books, and provide references and photocopies of articles which may be of interest to colleagues. These are alphabetically filed on the ward and are available to all staff and students, as well as directorate and trust colleagues. The articles are being placed on the computer data-base by the library access nurse. (Goddard 1996)

Local specialists

Local specialist knowledge has been utilised in the units in a variety of ways. For example, it may be the expertise of the leader that has been capitalised on. In some instances particular processes are used to share expertise, such as project supervision, where those with research skills have supported less experienced colleagues in developing the skills of project work. Another approach has been for individuals to focus on particular aspects of clinical and other work. One of the team members in the Day Ward NDU in Worthing has become the local expert in the management of lymphoedema. On Homeward NDU in Brighton a team member took a specific interest in wound care and has produced written material to help others both within and beyond the NDU.

Expertise of clinical leader

It was the clinical expertise of the leader of Annex NDU in the highly-specialised field of anorexia which led to the introduction of this nurse-led service. The clinical leader had spent many years working in a research team undertaking major follow-up studies with people who had had anorexia nervosa for varying lengths of time. She had also worked with the Eating Disorders Association for a number of years. She learnt that many people preferred, and did well, with outpatient care, and that there was no single treatment which was more successful than another for this group of patients. This has been essential to the life of the project, where the clinical leader has a consultant role to the team and other staff. By disseminating this knowledge to other members of the team, both formally and informally, the team has built up a body of knowledge which allows it to offer training and consultancy in a field where there is insufficient expertise to meet the clinical demand. (Annex NDU Annual Report 1994)

Practice and personal development through project supervision

One of the achievements of the John Radcliffe Hospital NDU has been practice and staff development through the supervision of clinical projects. The projects grew from practice and deal with issues which challenge or promote quality patient care. The experience of conducting these projects has been effective in developing inquiring practitioners whilst the completed studies enhance practice locally and act as a national resource. Examples are: the aromatherapy project (which focused on a survey of use and the related knowledge base); organisation of care project (aimed at auditing the nursing teams' practice of primary nursing); the bereavement booklet; and the professional needs of part-time staff (a project aimed at gaining insight into the integration of part-time nurses within their ward team, and at ascertaining their particular problems and needs). (Oxford Radcliffe Hospital Annual Report 1994–5)

Specialist link nurses

Link nurses have been developed in Bowthorpe NDU and across the trust for areas such as diabetes, nutrition, infection control, resuscitation, pain, continence, leg ulcer care and enhanced practice. They meet regularly and it is their responsibility to ensure safe practice, education and updating of the ward staff in and beyond the NDU. (Bowthorpe NDU Annual Report 1995)

Wound assessment link nurse

A primary nurse became the link nurse for wound management on Homeward NDU following a very successful period of time out to research the subject. Her booklet *Everything you wanted to know about wound management on Homeward but were afraid to ask* was followed by a wound assessment tool which she devised. (see Phelan *et al.* 1992) Along with the Waterlow Score and Sterling Pressure Sore Scale this is enclosed in every care plan to ensure all nurses have an easy-to-follow guide to assess the precise stage of healing of a wound. The tool encourages a holistic and reflective approach so that the choice of treatment relates to a particular wound at a particular stage of healing in one particular patient. The challenge now is to develop the tool as new research becomes available. This primary nurse is seen as an expert in the field by the unit and as the only ward-based nurse on the Brighton Health Care Wound Care Group, and is able to promote and receive new ideas from a position of clinical practitioner.

Library access nurse

Bowthorpe NDU has identified one member of the team as a library access nurse, to manage a resource room and maintain up-to-date research literature for nursing staff. Every two weeks a topic of nursing interest is selected and relevant information displayed. The nurse responds to requests from staff members for information and links with other departments and institutions (e.g. British Heart Foundation) to identify leaflets of value to patients and visitors. Student projects and assignments are catalogued and student welcome packs made available. (Bowthorpe Annual Report 1994)

Using skills of experts

Many nurses attend courses in order to gain new skills but find that they are not able to make best use of this knowledge when they return to practice. Through well-planned staff development such situations are unusual in NDUs. The first example given below demonstrates a creative way in which the skills of nurses working elsewhere in the trust have been used within the NDU in order to give them an opportunity to make use of their expertise.

Sessional work

The introduction of sessional work in the day-care unit of the Michael Flanagan NDU by team members and other trust personnel has been undertaken in order that they can make best use of the human resources and skills available to the organisation in a creative way. This has led to much greater interaction between day-care and inpatient service personnel and vastly increased the range of possibilities open to patients for treatment options. A policy on sessional work has been introduced across the trust, establishing individual access to becoming an associate consultant or sessional worker to the NDU. This is an important policy as the empowering nature of becoming involved has been formally and pragmatically encouraged (Sheehan 1994).

Developing new services

In many of the NDUs new services have been developed following a team member's concern for a specific patient problem which had not been adequately addressed. For example, in the Day Ward in Worthing one team member has developed skills in the management of lymphoedema and now provides a local specialist service for patients which is currently the subject

See also page 63

of research (Sitzia 1995). Similarly, the nurse-led enuresis service in Southampton has been created through concern for people with this problem and the development of the expertise of the nurse who initiated the work (Phillips 1995).

SUMMARY

Being able to account for practice to patients and clients and to employers means it is essential that we are able to explain the reasoning on which that practice is based. It must also be remembered that the sources of knowledge which are drawn on in making clinical decisions are not just taken from the more formal scientific research but also from personal meaning and acceptability to those concerned, the context in which care is given or received, and the moral dimension which is evident in all decision making. All of us have a duty to appraise critically our own work, be prepared to challenge and sometimes change our own practice, and to recognise the limits of our own knowledge as well as the expertise of others. There is no excuse for basing practice on folk-lore and tradition but neither should we jump onto a vogue band-wagon without good reason. It is essential to have an open and enquiring mind and a willingness to explore new options.

The examples which have been included in this section demonstrate some of the steps which nurses, midwives and health visitors have undertaken to challenge the status quo and increase the use of knowledge in practice. However, as you explore other areas in this directory it will become evident that seeking evidence is a fundamental component in many of the other sections. For example, there is an impact on the use of knowledge through the personal development of team members since it has helped those concerned to gain skills of critical appraisal. Similarly, evaluation of development work helps give insight into the efficacy of new ways of practising and in the research section specific activities which are seeking to increase our understanding of practice have been recorded.

Because of the wide public interest in the use of evidence in practice we have included practical examples in order to demonstrate some of the ways in which this issue has been addressed within the NDUs. In a wider context there is considerable literature available on the principles that are concerned with changing professional behaviour in relation to the use of evidence, and a few key references have been included as suggested further reading.

References & related reading

Allen M (1992) 'Pain management-influencing the nursing team' in Black G (1992) *Nursing Development Units Work in Progress* London, King's Fund

Bowthorpe *Annual Report* (1994) Norfolk and Norwich Healthcare NHS Trust

Bowthorpe *Annual Report* (1995) Norfolk and Norwich Healthcare NHS Trust

Boyd M, Brummell K, Billingham K, Perkins E (1993) *The Public Health Post at Strelley: An Interim Report* Strelley NDU Nottingham Community Trust

Chelsea and Westminster Intensive Care and NDU *Annual Report* July 1993–June 1994

Dickson R, Callum N (1996) 'Systematic Reviews: how to use the information' *Nursing Standard* 10(20) 32

Dutton J M, Grylls L, Goldstone L A (1991) *Accident and emergency nursing monitor: an audit of the quality of nursing care in hospital accident and emergency departments* Loughton, Gale Centre Publications

Kitson A (1990) *Quality Patient Care. The Dynamic Standard Setting System* Harrow, Scutari Press.

Gadd D (1995) *Information Technology* Cartmel NDU, Mental Health Services of Salford NHS Trust (also available on Internet – front sheet Cartmel NDU)

Gadd D, Colgan L, McFadden K (1995) *Research Based Care Plans: a Case Study of Research Use in Mental Health Nursing* Cartmel NDU, Mental Health Services of Salford NHS Trust

Goddard N (1996) *Everything you wanted to know about research but were afraid to ask* Bowthorpe Nursing Development Unit, Norfolk and Norwich Healthcare NHS Trust

Goldstone LA, Maselino Okai, C. V. (1986) *Senior monitor – an index of the quality of nursing care for senior citizens on hospital wards* Newcastle, Newcastle-upon-Tyne Polytechnic

Homeward Rehabilitation Unit (1991) *Standards Document* Homeward NDU, Brighton Healthcare Trust

Laxade S, Carney T (1992) *Standards for Orthopaedic Nursing* internal document, Newcastle, R.V.I. Hospital

Littlewood S, Saeidi S (1994) 'Therapeutic Mealtimes' *Elderly Care* 6(6) 20–21

Orem D E (1991) *Nursing – Concepts of Practice* (4th ed) New York, McGraw Hill

Oxford Radcliffe Hospital *Annual Report* 1994–5

Phelan P, Hawkey B, Sheppard B (1992) 'Wound Care: research alongside care' in Black G *Nursing Developments Work in Progress* London, King's Fund

Royal Liverpool and Broadgreen University Trust NDU (1995) *Final Report*

Sills E (1992) 'The Power Struggle' *Journal of Clinical Nursing* 2(1) 4

Sitzia J (1995) 'Volume Measurement in Lymphoedema Treatment: examination of formulae' *European Journal of Cancer Care* 4(1) 11–16

Stepney NDU *Annual Report* (1994)

Stocking B (1992) 'Promoting change in clinical practice in quality in health care' *Quality in Health Care* 1(1) 56–60

Truth Ward NDU *Annal Report* 1992–5, North Middlesex Hospital

Truth Ward NDU *Annual Report* 1993–4, North Middlesex Hospital

Vaughan B, Edwards M (1995) *Interface between Research and Practice* London, King's Fund

Waterworth S, Byrne C (1995) 'Benchmarking Quality Rules' *Nursing Management* 2(3) 13

Waterworth S (1995) 'Exploring the value of clinical nursing: the practitioner's perspective' *Journal of Clinical Nursing* 22(1) 13–17

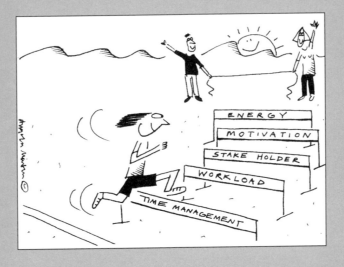

Part 3

DEVELOPMENTAL WORK

Development work, which here differs from more formal research activity, is a fundamental way of life in NDUs. By development work we mean activities which the units have undertaken to improve the services they offer patients or clients. This may mean the *use* of evidence in practice, an exploration of new roles, introducing new patterns of work organisation, or new services. The extent of activities is very wide-ranging and is based on local needs. What may be developmental for one unit may be common practice in another. For example, taking on new areas of technical work may be acceptable in a highly specialised area such as an intensive care unit but not in a general medical ward. Similarly, ideas which have been explored in one speciality may be new in another. Use of clinical supervision is not new to many nurses working in mental health or to midwives but its introduction in other areas is still in its infancy.

Despite these variations there appear to be characteristics which stimulate development work for all the NDUs. At the outset of this programme we explored this issue with a number of the clinical leaders, using a force-field analysis to elicit both the driving and constraining forces (Morrison 1992). Four features were common to all the participants, namely a fundamental humanistic value of the people to whom the service was offered; a belief that nursing had an important role to play in improving that service; the ability to think creatively and explore alternative options in response to a felt need, deficit or gap in the service; and the ability to act on initiative rather than wait for someone else to suggest what should be done. The needs rarely came from a formal theoretical perspective, despite exceptions, but from a deep concern that the current service was not meeting the needs of the patients adequately. The clinical leaders and their teams have taken action to solve problems.

Collating the development work undertaken by the NDUs over the past few years has, in itself, been rewarding in bringing to light just how much has been achieved. The skill of those concerned in managing change, over and above that demanded of such a turbulent health service, is a clear demonstration of just what can be achieved given the commitment and drive. Experience tells us that it is the getting going which is so challenging and that the small first steps, which look simple to the outsider, are as complex as the larger more visible developments. In reality, one feeds off the other and it is the inter-relationship of both large and small scale work which creates the turbulence of change.

Development work categories tend to overlap so, for convenience, we have divided this section into five broad parts related to user involvement, clinical services, organisation of care, roles, and theoretical perspectives. It has not been possible to include every activity and we would commend the individual reports of the units for more detail.

Involving Users

A great deal of the developmental work of the units is related to the users of the services – the patients, clients, their relatives and friends – and involving patients and their carers in decision-making has been central to their philosophy. These activities can be distinguished as those where information is sought from service users (and their carers), where patients or clients are given information, and situations where nursing practices involve the patients or clients.

Seeking patients' and clients' views

Information has been sought from clients, patients and their carers through a variety of different means, including traditional methods such as questionnaires and more novel approaches such as patient story-telling following discharge. Ways have also been explored for involving users in service provision, often through the development of groups, panels and forums.

Patient and family satisfaction

Chelsea and Westminster ICU NDU identified that the nursing staff needed to consider patient and family satisfaction with care in relation to primary nursing. This was in order to improve the service offered and to enable them to maintain the values of family-centred care. The difficulties of measuring patient and family satisfaction as a concept were recognised, particularly in the ICU patient group, as a large number of patients have decreased levels of consciousness for a significant period of their stay on the unit. Patient satisfaction was also identified as a trust objective for all areas of the hospital.

Six volunteers met in order to develop approaches to understanding the experiences of patients and families in ICU and to develop strategies to improve that experience. The intentions of the group were that patients and families would feel listened to and involved; staff would be assisted to build relationships; staff's awareness and understanding of the families' experience would be enhanced; areas for improvement would be identified and fed back into practice; and that others' awareness of what nurses do would be increased. Progress has included:

- An extensive literature search divided into four areas: patient satisfaction generally, patient satisfaction within ICU; family satisfaction, and the use of narratives in understanding the patient's experience
- The identification of potential research questions
- Preliminary work has been carried out interviewing relatives to explore their experience of the nursing care while they have a family member on the unit. (Chelsea and Westminster Intensive Care and NDU Annual Report 1994–5, Mills 1995)

See also page 105

User involvement: developing a satisfaction monitoring system for patients and relatives

Ashington (Ward 5) NDU has developed an approach to monitoring patient and family satisfaction with the aim of making it much easier for patients and relatives to express concerns or dissatisfaction at an early stage in the care process. A poster is displayed on the board above each patient's bed encouraging patients and relatives to make their concerns known to staff at an early stage. A patient and relative satisfaction sheet is available, together with a general comment/ suggestion sheet, in each patient's record folder which is located at the foot of the bed. Patients and relatives are encouraged to fill in the sheets to give a satisfaction rating of one to ten and comments before discharge, or to fill them in at home and return them by post. Any issues of concern raised by the patient or relatives whilst in hospital are dealt with by the relevant primary or associate nurse.

All completed satisfaction and comment sheets are reviewed at the monthly ward staff meeting which allows the team to learn issues of concern to patients and relatives, and to try to find solutions. It also provides positive feedback for the team which is important for morale and for keeping attention on the needs and views of patients.

The majority of comments have been very positive, with most satisfaction rating scores being eight or above. However, given the reluctance of most patients to criticise hospital staff (and nurses especially) what is more encouraging is the fact that patients and relatives are using the system to voice very real concerns about various aspects of the overall quality of the service and care.

For example, patients feel that they are getting a good quality service from nurses but they are concerned for the pressures which nurses are working under, and they desire more (not less) attention from them. (Ashington (ward 5) NDU Annual Report 1994)

Patient story-telling to generate quality improvement initiatives

One of the main projects of the John Radcliffe Hospital NDU was to develop a quality improvement programme which was responsive to the real concerns of patients as well as meeting the national agenda relating to consumerism and the efficacy of services. The unit felt that the use of questionnaires was limited since they are confined mainly to the areas defined by those designing them. As an alternative, an approach involving narratives was developed. This entailed patients recalling, about one month after discharge, their experiences whilst in hospital. Patients who agreed to participate were visited in their homes and invited to tell their own stories. The interviews, which were intentionally unstructured – though prompts were used – were taped and transcribed. The transcriptions were then subjected to a cognitive mapping process in order to produce a master map of indicators of good practice and quality improvement opportunities from the patients' perspectives. Areas for action included: getting into hospital, admission to the ward, hospital experiences (e.g. relationships, nights, visiting, contact with doctors) and discharge. From this information changes can be made which are of relevance to patients as indicators of good, and conversely, poor practice. (see Adair 1994, 1996)

Involving users

Stepney NDU set out to look specifically at how the unit could involve local people in the development work being undertaken by community nurses, and to explore replicable models for user involvement. Their particular concern was to engage local people in community health needs with a view to developing more sensitive provision. Several initiatives have also been undertaken to raise awareness about the lives of the residents. One in particular has been a collaborative activity with media students from a local college who, together with audio-visual assistance, have made a video in which four residents (two Bangladeshi and two white East Enders) give their accounts of life in the neighbourhood that include their health and housing needs.

This is shown to students and health workers to stimulate discussion about the population's requirements. (Stepney Nursing Development Unit 1993)

A follow-up video is in production entitled *Hundred Voices*. This will 'give 100 local people up to two minutes each to talk about their experiences of living in Stepney, and to say what one thing would make a difference to their health' (see Copperman and Morrison 1995). It will 'provide a platform for a chronologically and ethnically representative sample of community members to identify central issues for their own and their community's health' (Stepney Nursing Development Unit Annual Report 1994).

Similarly, Tameside and Glossop Mental Health NDU has introduced a system called CHAMP (Community and Hospital Advocacy for Mental Health Persons) which has been very effective in introducing and training clients as advocates for fellow clients. Advocates have focused on patients' rights, rather than providing alternative therapy services. The service has not only been therapeutic for the people involved but has had an impact on further service developments. Advocates have also been asked to support clients in other parts of the trust. (see Copperman and Morrison 1995)

Within Liverpool NDU enabling patients to feel they have more control is a particularly important aim, and the development of patient-controlled analgesia supports this idea. The unit is undertaking a study to compare the continuous infusion method of administering diamorphine with a patient-controlled analgesia (PCA) method. Data collected will be examined to determine whether using a PCA system improves pain control; entails decreased use of diamorphine; results in less side effects as measured by nausea and respiratory depression and so forth. Future areas for research will be identified. (Royal Liverpool NDU Annual Report 1994)

Users' groups

Within Michael Flanagan NDU, a users' group meets with an outside facilitator to explore and discuss client needs and service developments. This group does not confine its comments to the day centre itself, but has met with the chair of the trust board, the chief executive and other managers. One outcome from this work was a specific request for more support for adults who had suffered childhood abuse. This resulted in the introduction of a new service which was recognised in the 1995 *Nursing Times* 3 Ms awards (Holley 1996).

Homeward NDU set up a patients' forum following an action research project which highlighted many areas of concern patients had previously felt unable to discuss with staff. It was initiated and is still facilitated by a primary nurse, who meets with the patients fortnightly at the forum. Patients have instigated many small but important changes such as the delivery of newspapers, velcro on bed curtains to prevent them being accidentally opened when nurses are carrying out intimate care, quietening of noisy doors, and positioning of grab rails, as well as major changes such as individual pendants linked to the call-bell system so that patients can feel safe when alone in the garden or sitting room if they wish. This has involved managers of catering, for example, being invited to the forum and for some it was their first face-to-face meeting with patients.

As well as promoting rehabilitation the forum has been a very powerful way of auditing quality. It has given nurses the unique opportunity to address issues which have previously remained unnoticed and is yet another move towards a patient-centred unit. (Clarke and Sheppard 1992)

Carers' panel

Southport NDU identified a need to find out what problems carers had and what support they required. They set up a panel of carers so they could have their own voices heard and take part in decision-making alongside other lay people – such as members of voluntary organisations – and health service workers. The panel raised many issues and five formed the focus of initial efforts:

- developing a teaching programme for carers
- developing a better understanding of medications
- publishing a booklet containing information needed by carers
- developing a 24-hour help line
- improving respite care facilities

The work instigated by the carers' panel has been evaluated by an independent researcher using semi-structured interviews. During each interview the carers felt the original points they identified were still important and all the carers considered that the panel was a good idea which had helped them. In order to overcome the problem that the panel was limited to those people who could attend the meetings, staff of the unit decided to supplement this work with visits to some carers in their own homes. (Horner 1992)

Providing information

Ensuring that patients and clients have access to information is an essential part of care if they are to have some control and become involved in decision-making about their own health. Ways of ensuring that information is shared include such activities as the introduction of information centres and groups, patient-held Filofaxes and the establishment of patient-centred working such as named nurses and self-medication systems.

Family information centre

The Child Health Directorate in conjunction with the Southampton Children's Outpatient Department NDU is developing a Centre for Health Information and Promotion (CHIP), the aim of which 'is to provide specialist materials for carers and children to help them understand and cope with health and illness-related family concerns' (Glasper *et al.* 1995). The NDU family-information nurse, a new role, is vital to this development. Underpinning the setting up of the CHIP is the concept of advocacy and the belief that information giving is one of the prime factors in patient empowerment. The CHIP will offer a range of services from traditional family-information leaflets to sophisticated telephone helpline support. In addition it will undertake trials of a CD-ROM-generated patient-information system. Evaluation of the centre will be an integral feature.

Friendship group

Worthing NDU has set up a Friendship Group for patients, ex-patients and their relatives, offering support and sharing for all those in need by people who have been through similar experiences. Volunteers are happy to visit patients if neccessary. The group also provides practical resources such as televisions and video recorders for wards. Many patients continue to attend for long periods of time and willingly offer their support to those who are new to the service, giving them a feeling of purpose and worth and an opportunity to contribute to the unit as well as to receive care. (Worthing Day Ward NDU Annual Report 1993–4)

Young carers project

Andover NDU has set up a young carers project to increase awareness and provide a support service for young people who have caring responsibilities in their homes. The aim of the project has been:

- to disseminate information to children
- to raise awareness amongst professionals on how to identify and be aware of a child who may be a carer of an adult at home
- to identify the specific issues these children might have and try to meet their needs

Action taken so far has included information folders for young carers, a multi-agency workshop for professionals, posters for schools, a painting competition and a market stall as well as a helpline. (Andover Annual Report 1994)

Patient Filofax

Bowthorpe NDU has pioneered a patient Filofax system, in the form of a small ring-binder which enables patients to go home with a complete personal record of treatments, drugs, special diets and exercise programmes. Space is also available for patients to make notes of symptoms or concerns which they may wish to discuss with a health-care worker. Extensive work has been undertaken with community staff, and meetings have been held with GP practices, locality managers, community professionals and the Care Group, to ensure involvement and co-operation. A random sample of 50 GPs was sent a draft copy of the Patient Information Pack for comments prior to its use and a small group of 15 patients has since taken part in a pilot study which is showing positive results. For example, one patient is now able to provide information about her new medication to the community team and another has found keeping a record of symptoms very helpful when meeting health-care workers. (Goddard 1996)

Introduction of named nurse concept

Southampton Children's Outpatient Department NDU believes that the children's nurse should be available for the family – a family advocate – and this aim has been pursued through introduction of the named nurse concept. A named children's nurse is identified for each clinic and families are presented with specially-designed business cards to enable them to contact her following consultation. This may be several days later when they have had time to evaluate concerns and identify their questions. The nurses have become experts in specific aspects of care through working regularly in scheduled clinics. This has also led to the introduction of nurse-led clinics where outpatient nurses with paediatric expertise are a regular face with whom the family can feel relaxed. They believe that this change is working well, providing the families with more information, helping towards a more friendly and welcoming department, and enabling the nurse to get to know regular attenders at clinics. (Lowson 1995)

Self-medication and compliance

For many years Homeward NDU has promoted self-medication programmes for selected patients and has seen excellent results in terms of safe administration of drugs on discharge, improved self-esteem and moves towards independence. One of the primary nurses decided to take this development one step further and has linked with the ward pharmacist (who is also a community pharmacist) to help promote compliance following discharge. They have formalised what was a vague and inconsistent system by ensuring that support and resources are available across the hospital and community trusts for patients and carers when the nurses have identified problem areas prior to discharge. Chemists have been found, for example, who will deliver medication, provide non-childproof bottles and identification codes, and patients and carers are now contacted after discharge to ensure that all is well. (Homeward NDU Annual Report 1992)

Client and patient-focused new practices

Users' interests have been the focus of new nursing practice in many of the units. This has ranged from a whole service revolving round user needs (as in the case of the ASHA project outlined below) to particular processes such as bedside handovers, through to personal relationships and the whole philosophy of units such as the examples from Witney and Glenfield NDUs below.

ASHA project

The ASHA project has been a collaborative venture between Stepney NDU and the ASHA (Bangladeshi for 'Hope') Asian Women's Group. It was established to provide more accessible preventive health-care to the predominantly Bangladeshi population of Tower Hamlets, and began with the setting up of a drop-in weekly clinic supported by a health visitor/ Bangladeshi link worker. This has greatly increased service uptake and rates of developmental assessment as well as providing opportunity for support and increasing awareness of the services which are available. It has also helped to increase awareness of the specific health-care needs of this group of women.

One of the areas of women's concerns related to infant feeding, and through the group, it was suggested that a more participatory approach to supporting weaning, grounded in the beliefs and perspectives of community members, could offer a more appropriate way forward. On this basis an application was successfully made to the National Dairy Council/Nursing Standard Research Award to carry out an action research project to investigate and support healthy weaning. This funding has been used to appoint a Bangladeshi research worker to undertake outreach work and facilitate discussion of health beliefs around weaning among inter-generation groups of community members. (Buxton 1993)

Another aspect of the ASHA project has been the link with the Community Arts Team so that a group of Bangladeshi women can work in facilitated discussion groups on an embroidered hanging on the theme of healthy eating. This hanging will form part of the National Textile Project's exhibition at the Victoria and Albert Museum. (Stepney NDU Annual Report 1994, James 1993)

Bedside handover linked to patient empowerment

Bowthorpe NDU has used the bedside handover to help patients become more involved in their treatment. Evaluation of the handover has revealed a number of issues, including the importance of the clinical leader's personality and her ability to delegate to the staff in ensuring the effectiveness of handover as a means of giving power to patients. Early evaluation also highlighted the point that not all patients wish to have so much involvement, seeing the role of the nurse and other staff as the 'authority' in their care and such views are taken into account in current practice. (Watkins and Theis 1993, Chadwick 1996)

West Dorset NDU, too, has been concerned about patient reporting. In an effort to increase patient participation and involvement in their care, the unit used action-centred research to move from nurse-dominated and office-centred handovers to patient-centred events located with the patients at their bedside. Outcomes have indicated that bedside handovers can improve and sustain effective nurse-patient communication. Patients showed increased satisfaction at being involved in care and increased their knowledge of care and treatments. (Waight 1992)

Handovers have also been replaced by the use of care plans with patient involvement at Seacroft (wards V and W) NDU and these practices are widespread throughout NDUs. (Wallum 1995)

Personal relationships

The East Berkshire NDU was concerned that people with learning disability had limited understanding of personal relationships, with the opportunity to develop this area of their lives. With support from the trust they established a development programme with evaluation of clients' knowledge and behaviour before and after the sessions. A sex education worker for men is now employed within the team, indicating trust-wide support for such work with people with learning disabilities. This work also received acknowledgement in the *Nursing Standard* Awards of 1995. (Morton 1995)

Making choices

Denying people the opportunity to make choices is to deny their right to individuality. The work on choice at the Witney NDU (a community-based service working with adults with a learning disability) began with the absence of a bottle of tomato sauce. This posed the question: How would you feel if in your own home you did not have the opportunity to make a choice as fundamental as whether or not you could have tomato sauce on or with your chips? The realisation that basic choices were not being afforded to people with learning disabilities underpinned much of the work of the unit. The Choice project was conducted over a two-year period. Activity flow charts were used to measure levels of choice in the home environment and ways in which choice could be increased were identified and piloted. For example, ways were sought of offering choice of flavourings with food, of television and radio programmes and of bath and bed times. In some instances this did entail risk-taking when, for example, one client with poor sight wished to cross a busy road unaccompanied, raising important questions about individual's rights to freedom. The study concluded that the greater the choice people have in their own lives, the more control they have, and that this leads to a better chance of attaining a higher quality of life. (Shephard and Garbett 1994, Sheppard 1994)

Self-care

Self-care, based on the work of the nurse theorist Dorothea Orem (1991), has been the underlying philosophy behind all development work at Glenfield NDU. The philosophy is based on a belief that we all have the right to care for ourselves whenever possible with self-determination about what we wish to achieve. It is around these beliefs that the development activities at Glenfield have been planned. The team have focused on ways to help patients become more empowered by bringing control and choice into their lives. For example, the use of self-medication is now well established as is the patient education programme. They also believe that if self-care is to go beyond rhetoric then it is continuity of care which is critical; this has led to the development work they have undertaken with primary nursing. (Furlong 1995, 1996)

Clinical Services

While all the work which has been included in this publication has, as an underlying purpose, the improvement of clinical care for patients, the activities within this section are the ones which have a direct rather than an indirect outcome. Inevitably, this is one of the largest parts of the directory and it has been subdivided into sections concerned with independent nurse-led initiatives, specific services, generic services, and organisational strategies. There is some overlap between these headings and, as is the case with other entries, each one must be viewed in the wider context of a whole service.

Developing an independent service

Some units have directed their attention to the establishment of a new service which is fundamental to the central purpose of their work. These initiatives involve not only the development of specialist skills in, for example, eating disorders, rehabilitation or therapeutic nursing, but also major work in negotiating with multi-professional colleagues as well as revising organisational and policy issues. The examples given below highlight steps which have been taken to introduce such services.

Establishment of a service for people with anorexia

In order to extend the work begun by the clinical leader for people with anorexia in Annex NDU and set up by a team of specialist nurse practitioners offering a nurse-led service, complex negotiations were required with medical and managerial colleagues, taking into account both clinical and organisational issues. Long delays occurred before the service could be established (which required considerable perseverance), but motivation was maintained by a commitment to the needs of this client group and belief in the efficacy of the treatment. Skills were developed in business planning, contracting, and change management. (see Halek *et al.* 1995, Cohen 1994) Within the past year the nurse-led service has split from the medically-led eating disorders service and now receives direct referrals from local general practitioners and psychiatrists, other health authorities and clients themselves.

Introduction of a new nurse-led in-service

At a time when there was considerable pressure on medical beds in the acute hospital Byron NDU offered an alternative nurse-led in-patient service to the trust. It was aimed at a clearly-defined group of patients who were medically stable but still required intensive nursing in order to gain maximum independence and quality of life. The thinking behind this plan was not only to provide care for this group's needs but also to relieve some of the pressure on the acute medical beds. To begin with steps were taken to develop clinical assessment skills of the nurses; to agree admission and discharge protocols and referral mechanisms; to arrange non-urgent medical cover through a part-time general practitioner; to agree emergency cover and so forth. The development of skills in physical assessment alongside relevant documentation, was important in ensuring the competence of the staff and the safety of the patients.

Patients who fit the criteria for admission to the unit are transferred as soon as possible after their medical condition has stabilised. Authority for management of care is transferred to the primary nurse who is in contact with other members of the health-care team and can arrange discharge as necessary. A major study to assess the impact of this service on patient outcomes is under way. It has recently been agreed to increase the number of nurse-led beds within the trust and expand the nurse-led service. (see Evans and Griffiths 1994)

Rehabilitation nursing

Homeward NDU's early work was based on research on the nursing role and function in rehabilitation. Now work has concentrated on providing a more comprehensive programme of rehabilitation for patients. The multi-professional team is well-established and, despite changes in personnel over the past year, nurses have taken on more nursing therapy sessions with their patients. The effect has been dramatic for many individuals and in some cases determined early discharge and a much improved outcome. This work is being monitored informally at present; it is hoped to formalise a study soon. (Sheppard 1994)

Setting up a midwifery-led unit

Royal Bournemouth Hospital NDU has set up a midwifery-led unit for low-risk women after a campaign in the early nineties to keep a local maternity service open rather than transfer care to the larger hospital in nearby Poole.

To achieve this the unit had to consider both organisational and clinical issues including:

- criteria to identify high- and low-risk women
- probable number of low-risk deliveries per year
- operational principles, clinical facilities and equipment
- maternity staff establishment
- development for the midwives
- preparation of women and client-held obstetric records
- preparation of GPs
- philosophy of care and objectives
- policies and standing orders
- cost

The work of this unit was established prior to the *Changing Childbirth* report (1993) but fulfils many of its requirements. Since opening, work has continued to develop many further aspects of the service. A report has been produced to help other midwives plan and establish such units. (Husbands and Thomas 1994)

Open referral system

An open referral system has been operated by Michael Flanagan NDU where referrals can be made directly to the day unit from community staff and clients without having to gain access via the psychiatrist. This has led to a substantial increase in the number of clients who can be supported by the service as well as making much fuller use of the range of skills among the team members. The service has continued to maintain its commitment to consultant staff referring from within the organisation. Both inpatient clients and those from the community can now access care in the day unit. (Sheehan 1994)

See also page 24

Development of a cardiac support group

Ashington (ward 5) NDU felt there was a need to give those with heart disease and their families more support (The incidence of coronary heart disease in the north-east is extremely high). Feedback from patient satisfaction forms, formal complaints, and informal feedback, showed that people felt they did not always receive the attention, information and emotional support they needed. Nurses from the NDU, coronary care and medical units came together with a dietician and a physiotherapist to form a cardiac support group, called Your Heart & You – Support Group. The group has devised a booklet for people who have suffered a heart attack entitled Your Heart and You which contains advice and information on medication, reducing risk factors, and a contact number and an invitation to join the support group. In the meetings, discussion has proved to be the most valuable aspect, when group members can talk about their experiences, or speak confidentially to one of the health-care professionals present. A fund-raising event was organised by a key member of the group, a bank account was opened, and they have since applied for charitable status. As a result of this local people have a cardiac support group which they are now organising and running themselves. (Ashington (ward 5) Annual Report 1993–4)

Specific clinical services and practices

A major aim of the units is to provide specific clinical services. Here there is a wide range of topics, including traditional services, with a new nurse-led orientation as well as complementary therapies such as aromatherapy. In addition, new roles have been developed and existing roles enlarged. The range of topics offers an exciting insight into the many ways in which nurses are expanding the care they offer to patients and clients.

Nurse-led enuresis clinic

Southampton Children's Outpatient Department NDU has a belief in the importance of nurse-led clinics and several have been introduced, one of which has provided an enuresis service. Traditionally children with enuresis have been referred to the outpatient department yet many were found to have no organic cause for the problem. The management strategies of each consultant varied, but many children were given only limited further support. A senior staff nurse in the unit felt that these children and their parents needed more help as well as specific support and guidance. Such care related more to nursing than medical skills, which has led to the development of the nurse-led clinic.

Guidelines were produced about how the clinic would be managed. Once patients are referred, nurses have the autonomy to obtain a detailed history of the problem and make their own clinical assessment. Subsequent management is based on the individual needs of the child drawing on a range of knowledge about different regimes which have proved helpful. Each patient is seen by the consultant within six months of their first appointment with the clinic. The unit nurse now acts as the link person between the hospital and community-based enuresis clinics and shared guidelines are in use.

Within three months of opening, the clinic was managing 34 children with new referrals weekly. Treatments which had not been offered previously are being introduced and audit of the clinical outcomes is under way. The success of the nurse-led clinic is judged by the amount of referrals received and the support for the service from both the patients and medical colleagues. This clinic was the forerunner of other nurse-led clinics such as the service for children with asthma. (Phillips 1995)

Well Leg project

Stepney NDU has set up the Well Leg project to give people with leg ulcers high quality research-based care to raise the awareness within the local community of the need to treat leg ulcers, and to develop systems of quality assurance for leg ulcer treatment of local people. A questionnaire incorporating these aims was used to ascertain the interest of the district nurses and a series of workshops run to develop knowledge and motivation. Measurements of cost-effectiveness and health outcomes have been incorporated into the project evaluation. A short-stretch compression bandaging system is being compared with a four-layer bandaging system, and healing rates are being monitored to provide a measurement which could be incorporated into a future outcomes-based care package.

The project has also led to the production of nursing standards for leg ulcer assessment, treatment and prevention and it is proposed that a district-wide link-nurse group for leg ulcer management is established in the locality.

In addition a users' group has been formed for women who have, or have recovered from, this problem. Nursing staff have found this a valuable way of gaining insight into their feelings and experiences of living with leg ulcers. The women gained knowledge and support from each other, and learned how to work with nurses to improve the service. Plans include further group work to produce an information leaflet; awareness-raising campaigns; further training workshops; implementation of the standards and research into the effects of the environment on healing rates. (Stepney NDU Annual Report 1994)

Lymphoedema service

Worthing NDU runs a specialist lymphoedema service in the form of a clinic which is nurse-initiated and nurse-led, with patients being referred by GPs, consultants, district nurses and physiotherapists. They aim to treat four new patients a month. A clinical nurses specialist who has undertaken training in this aspect of care has responsibility for running the service with support from other colleagues. The service is unique in the geographical area of the NDU, and the number of referrals is increasing as colleagues from other professions learn about it. The work is complemented by a sequential trial of two lymphoedema treatments which has been initiated on the ward. Since one treatment regime takes half an hour and the other two hours the outcome of this study will have considerable impact on the day-to-day running of the service. (Sitzia 1995)

Hickman Line project

Nurses in Worthing NDU have also completed an information booklet *The care and use of the Hickman Line*, which is used widely in GP surgeries and hospitals in the surrounding area as well as locally in the trust. The booklet has helped patients gain a better understanding of what to expect when they commence their treatment regimes. A video is being produced to augment the booklet, showing patients having treatments and procedures, with a demonstration of the Hickman Line. The team are also negotiating to extend their services to include removal of Hickman Lines, a procedure which has previously been the task of medical staff, a restriction which causes additional delays for patients. (Worthing Day Ward Annual Report 1993–4)

The EMERGE project

The Michael Flanagan NDU has launched EMERGE (formerly known as SCOPE). This is a service provided in partnership with the trust and the non-statutory sector. It gives support to individuals who have been sexually abused in the past and is aimed at exploring ways in which they can learn to live with their experiences. EMERGE is now run as a free-standing service in the trust with direct access for clients. This development was recognised as an award winner in the *Nursing Times*/3Ms 1995 programme. (Holly 1996).

Nutrition

Southport NDU identified the problem of nutritional deficiencies in elderly people, but concluded that they were not doing enough to detect, correct and prevent them in their own elderly patients. They introduced a slightly modified Nutrition Assessment Checklist (originally designed by the Nutrition Advisory Group for the Elderly), as a user-friendly assessment tool and as part of a flexible health promotion programme to meet the special needs of their patients and carers. The checklist highlights the potential problems caused by drastic weight changes as well as alerting nurses and patients to the relationship between vitamin supplements and certain medical conditions, leading to a need for specific nutrients in the diet. In addition, food preferences can be taken into account. The benefits are manifold. For example, it has enhanced nurses' knowledge of nutrition and its relationship to the health of the patients in general; it has highlighted the role of the nurse in health education; and it has provided more specific information to those caring for particular patients about their nutritional status. It has also encouraged the unit to explore the use of a more comprehensive tool which takes into account nutritional, psychological, socio-economic and medical factors to improve care for the elderly. (see McGuire 1992)

Therapeutic mealtimes

Seacroft (wards V and W) NDU has recognised the social importance of mealtimes for their patients, believing that as mental health nurses they could contribute to the improvement of a therapeutic environment. Data were collected by observation and questionnaires. (Two questionnaires were developed – one for staff, one for patients.) The observation form was used to assess four main areas: patients' choices at mealtimes; the environment; interaction between patients and nurses; the general atmosphere. The main objectives of the work have been to improve the quality of mealtimes, increase choices available to patients, raise self-awareness of staff and encourage socialising at mealtimes. A standard has also been developed against which the quality of this service can be assessed. (see Littlewood and Saeidi 1994)

Self-medication programmes

Truth Ward NDU introduced a self-medication programme which showed that their previous practice disempowered patients in many ways and has since led to a search for other methods of increasing patient control such as the introduction of a cardiac rehabilitation programme. On average, a fifth of all patients are now on self-medication programmes at any one time, and the aim of the unit is to increase this figure. This project, while focusing on a single area of care, has been a significant stimulus for further work influencing the perceptions and actions of the clinical team. (Truth Ward NDU 1995)

Maintaining the highest degree of independence for patients has been a priority for the Newcastle NDU, and they believe that patients in managing their own medication is one aspect of this. A pilot study, targeted at elderly people who are not confused or disoriented, has been conducted to assess the interest in self-administration. The process has been evaluated using an action research approach which formed part of an MSc dissertation (Rees 1995).

The West Dorset NDU looked at patients' needs for communication and information about their medications, together with increased patient involvement in their care, and concluded that a system of self-administration of medicines was appropriate. Led by a primary nurse, a protocol was drawn up in collaboration with the hospital's pharmacist. Issues such as storage and consent were addressed. Further developments in this area have been a patient-held booklet and record chart. General information about taking medicines is included in the booklet, as well as space for recording information about specific medicines. The booklets, which are the property of the patient and can be taken home, have also been found to be useful for patients not self-medicating. The scheme not only involves patients, but raises nurses' awareness and develops skills in giving information about medicines generally. A follow-up audit of discharged patients who were self-medicating on the unit has been undertaken and a report will be available shortly.

As part of their overall research programme Glenfield NDU has undertaken a study to explore patients' understanding of their medications, comparing those who were taking their own medication with those who did not. (Furlong 1996)

See also page 126

Continence assessment

Continence assessment has been another project in the Newcastle NDU. All patients admitted to the unit with an identified continence problem are assessed using an Assessment of Urinary Incontinence standard. A systematic approach is then used to plan and implement a management strategy involving both nursing and medical expertise. This retention of urine has been identified as a major cause of incontinence, and a protocol, validated by medical colleagues, has been produced to raise awareness of the problem particularly with orthopaedic patients. The principles and approach used have now been disseminated across the trust, and have influenced the development of a Trust Continence Advisor post. (Royal Victoria Infirmary NDU Annual Review 1992–3)

Named nurse

The team at Weston Park (Sheffield) NDU felt that they could improve their approach to the named nurse concept. Their first step was to set a standard and agree criteria before and after implementation of the changes which they found made nurses more aware of their responsibilities as named nurses. For example, co-ordination of the patient's discharge had previously been undertaken by the senior nurse but is now recognised as the responsibility of the named nurse. The audit has also shown that nurses now explain the concept of named nursing more effectively to patients. (Denison 1994)

Aromatherapy and massage

The use of aromatherapy and massage as supportive therapies is quite widespread amongst the NDUs, many of whom have given one or more of the team the opportunity to gain formal training in this skill. For example in Seaford NDU this service is offered to the elderly mentally infirm clients at night to provide calm and comfort. Similarly, the service has been developed at Weston Park within the oncology unit and local evaluation has been carried out in the intensive care unit in Brighton Healthcare. (*Nursing Standard News* 1992) Other examples follow below.

In the Seacroft NDU, following a period of training, two members of staff are able to offer massage with base and essential oils as a form of anxiety management to patients experiencing anxiety problems. Primary nurses refer their patients to the trained nurse and if appropriate she will undertake massage sessions. Both she and the patient keep notes on how they feel the sessions went. The nurse has produced questionnaires for patients to complete as a means of monitoring its effectiveness, and a formal review of the service, with the help of the nurse researcher, is anticipated for the future. Early indications suggest mixed reactions to the massage from participants, but it does appear to have enhanced patient confidence and self-image, encouraged self-responsibility and increased motivation. (see Fascione 1995)

See also page 40

A survey of 13 medical and surgical wards within the host hospital was undertaken by John Radcliffe Hospital NDU as a supervised clinical project. The results indicated that aromatherapy practice was widespread and popular with nursing staff. However, practice standards and protocols were absent; personal knowledge mainly guided its utilisation and evaluation did not generally occur. Recommendations for a review of practice were made, entailing the temporary cessation of aromatherapy until such time that competency and safety could be ensured. (Oxford Radcliffe Hospital NDU Annual Report 1995–6)

Sheffield Occupational Health NDU has also been exploring the use of aromatherapy in high-stress work areas and some members of the team have had specific training. Working initially with the local fire and rescue service control room staff, the aims of the project are several:

- to establish the presence and degree of stress in the group
- to provide aromatherapy as one means of coping in the management of stress
- to enable promotion of well-being in the workplace
- to ensure information is available

A psychologist is co-ordinating evaluation of the project which is being done by discussion and the completion of a questionnaire by all individuals receiving the treatment and advice. Work has also begun on a code of practice for the use of aromatherapy in the city council. (see Sheffield Occupational Health NDU Annual Report 1994–5)

Development of art therapy

Michael Flanagan NDU has used art therapy, in conjunction with a theory of management of consequences, as a treatment option for patients. This project has been undertaken by a team member who was released from day-to-day practice through his clinical fellowship scheme (Vaughan and Edwards 1995) in order to have time to work on the development. He can now offer a well-developed service with very encouraging results for patients who have not responded well to other forms of treatment. (Dodd 1994)

Reminiscence work

Seacroft NDU has recognised the importance of reminiscence for elderly patients with a range of mental health needs including dementia. A reminiscence room has been set up in the unit which is decorated and furnished in the style of the 1930s-1940s. Reminiscence work has been undertaken with small groups of patients to offer people admitted to the ward more opportunities to socialise and build relationships. Vague themes are introduced by the staff, but the general conversation, social contact and tea-drinking has its own momentum. This work has been examined to identify whether conducting formal reminiscence sessions within a period environment had any specific therapeutic gain. The groups comprised five to nine individuals and met once or twice a week. Different environments, including the reminiscence room, were used to enable comparison. At the conclusion of the groups (18 patients in total took part), a semi-structured interview was conducted to gain insight into the experience of participants. The results appeared to support a positive link between a themed room and the reminiscence process. The period setting of the room seemed to facilitate the recall of memories from that time; however, it also allowed recall from periods other than that represented by the setting. The conclusion was that environment is significant in reminiscence activity, but the period setting seems to be of less importance than the comfort and informality of the room. (see Gilley and David 1995)

Snoezelen

Seacroft (wards Vand W) NDU have been using Snoezelen (which was developed in Holland) to provide people who have sensory and learning disabilities with appropriate relaxation and leisure facilities. It consists of pleasurable sensory experiences generated in an atmosphere of trust and relaxation. The experiences are arranged to stimulate primary senses without the need for intellectual activity. Trust and relaxation are encouraged by a non-directive or enabling approach being adopted by the helper or carer. At Seacroft the unit is working with three of the more disabled individuals using a more structured approach, and their behaviour is being monitored before, during and after the session. After initial sessions the three individuals appeared more alert and interested in their surroundings. Special environments have been created in many areas (home, hospitals etc.) and the aim of the unit is to develop its own multisensory room for use by its clients. (Seacroft (wards V and W) NDU Second Annual Report)

Expansion of services

Expansion of the services which nurses offer to patients and clients has been a common feature of many NDUs. For example, in Royal Bournemouth Hospital NDU some of the new services which have been developed include:

- school visits by midwives to teach teenagers about the midwife's role
- single mothers' groups for single mothers and pregnant teenagers (Dunford 1995)
- extended skills in cannulation

Much of their project work has also included expansion of the services previously offered including evaluation of water-births, teaching of junior doctors and support with breast feeding. (Royal Bournemouth Hospital NDU Annual Report 1995)

Introduction of play therapist

The introduction of formalised therapeutic play in the Southampton Children's Outpatient Department NDU has given the entire multi-disciplinary team an opportunity to learn new skills. The play specialist, appointed to the NDU, has helped create a play environment acceptable to all age groups and facilitates both normal and diversional play. Play introduces normality into a strange setting which can markedly lessen the impact of pain and anxiety. The play specialist and, through her guidance, the nursing staff, can allow the child to work through negative feelings and fears, thus enabling the outpatient visit to become a positive experience. This has been particularly successful for children with needle phobias. Another project has been that of joint working between a senior staff nurse and the play specialist to plan a preparation club for children who are undergoing Micturating Cysto-Urethrogram Examination. In addition the NDU play specialist is working with another play specialist to establish a sibling support group for diabetic and cystic fibrosis patients. (see Lowson 1995)

Developing a generic service

Rather than concentrate on a specific clinical service development, some units have focused on services which have broader aims. Sheffield Occupational Health NDU is a particular example where an over-riding concern for stress in the workplace has led to three programmes, illustrated in the first entry below. Other units have initiated services within the NDU which are now available more widely that highlight the generic nature of much nursing work.

Stress management

The main thrust of the work of the Sheffield Occupational Health NDU has been stress management and this became an umbrella for other endeavours within the unit such as the use of different therapeutic methods to alleviate stress. A stress working party has been set up to look at organisational factors. Evaluation of stress management courses has been part of the remit of this working party.

Redundancy programmes In addition, the unit has programmes to cope with compulsory redundancy and to tackle causes of occupational stress. Faced with possible compulsory redundancy in the city council, an Occupational Health Nurse (OHN) worked with other members of the personnel and education department to provide support and training schemes for staff who might be affected. The sessions were multi-disciplinary and considered many aspects of redundancy, with the OHN concentrating on the health aspects and the depression caused by job loss. The seminars were run in schools faced with closure that academic year. Although they were difficult to operate because of the content of the sessions and the emotions raised there was a high degree of satisfaction for those involved. They did, however, generate an increased workload for the OHN as people came to realise that they were suffering from stress and related problems. This identified a need for stress management training for head-teachers in schools in the area and this is now being introduced. (see Sheffield Occupational Health NDU Annual Report 1993–1994)

Counselling service Furthermore, Sheffield Occupational Health NDU has set up a specialised workplace-based counselling service for employees. Clients can be referred to this service by the OHN who has responsibility for the area in which they work. The project is an essential requirement in reducing the long-term impact of problems experienced by employees and the unavoidable delay in receiving appropriate help through more traditional resources. Individuals are seen on a pre-determined number of occasions and the outcomes measured. This service has now exceeded its weekly time allocation due to demand and has been allocated a full-time occupational health nurse. (see Sheffield Occupational Health NDU Annual Report 1994–1995).

Introduction of stroke care team and cardiac rehabilitation service

Truth Ward NDU has, after considerable planning, succeeded in establishing a stroke care team. There has been a high level of commitment to the service and members of the team feel that it has a direct impact on the care of stroke patients within the hospital. The organisation of the team needs further development and there is a plan to audit standards.

They have also introduced a cardiac rehabilitation service for the patients. This is well attended by up to 12 people per session and feedback from patients is very positive though, owing to increased numbers and lack of resources on the ward, some organisational problems have been encountered.

A comprehensive cardiac rehabilitation service, including an exercise plan, is now offered to patients following myocardial infarction, coronary artery bypass graft and angioplasty. (Truth Ward NDU 1995)

Supportive therapy unit

Liverpool NDU has had an interest in complementary therapies for some time and has recognised the need to make this service available to both patients and staff throughout the trust. Talks were held to establish a service for one afternoon each week in the out-patient department where staff who had gained qualification in massage and the use of essential oils would offer treatment. Referrals are now received from medical staff as well as self-referrals of colleagues and an additional session is being offered. Questionnaires given to users produced very positive feedback. The NDU team, in conjunction with Phoenix Development (the training and development department of the trust) also offer a course to 'heighten awareness and develop both practical and theoretical skills in complementary approaches to health care'. The course which spans 15 weeks has recently been validated through the Lancashire College of Nursing and Health Studies as an ENB N17 programme. (Royal Liverpool and Broadgreen University Trust NDU 1995)

Patient education

Like many other units the Royal Victoria Infirmary NDU has prepared a patient education package, in this instance for individuals attending the Orthopaedic out-patients department. To promote this activity a member of the NDU staff took a Certificate in Health Education which was part of a much wider staff-development programme.

Similarly, as part of the overall philosophy for self-care Glenfield NDU has worked on improving the information and learning opportunities offered to patients; this has been a major aim of their activities. (Glenfield NDU 1995)

In Stepney NDU a video has been made to help both staff and members of the local population gain insight into the lives and health-care needs of people living in Tower Hamlets (Stepney Nursing Development Unit 1993), and Worthing NDU have also prepared specialist material for patients who will be living for some time with a Hickman Line.

See also page 65

Organisational strategies

In developing particular clinical services, units have used different strategies and systems. Sometimes the aim has been to encompass the whole environment or a major aspect of the unit's work. At other times the approach used strategies such as dementia care mapping, educational and supervisory activities or specific tools. The emphasis has been to look at a range of different issues which will directly or indirectly improve working practice.

Improving the therapeutic environment

A major objective for Anston Ward NDU at Rampton Hospital has been to improve the therapeutic environment for both the patients and staff. This work was tackled in a number of different ways including:

- a dramatic decrease in the use of seclusion as a means of controlling unacceptable behaviour following reappraisal of traditional work practices where concern for nurses' safety led to custodial regimes; changing staff attitudes to seclusion; changes in power balances and attention to patient-centred care; and the introduction of a women's group for staff and patients to deal with gender issues without fear of prejudice.
- continuity of care, the introduction of the named nurse and care planning. Early research demonstrated room for improvement in all these areas and steps are now under way to bring about changes.
- the use of critical incidents to identify the range of approaches to problem solving and staff feelings about these approaches. The data were subjected to content analysis which confirmed the stressful nature of the work but also identified new ways in which problems could be resolved. In most cases the difficulty lay not in knowing *what* to do but in *how* to do it. Changes have included the introduction of clinical supervision and alterations to the structure and timing of staff support groups.
- establishing links with Annex NDU to promote work on eating disorders, a common problem with this patient group. This link has helped the Anston team to gain skills in helping patients manage some of their complex difficulties with eating.
- auditing of care plans as a starting point for moving to more individualised programmes for the patient.

Other areas of work include skills development for care assistants, an exploration of the interactions between the providers and recipients of care, the use of multidisciplinary documentation and the introduction of therapeutic touch. Each of these initiatives is subject to internal evaluation. (Anston Ward NDU 1993)

Bridging therapy

The main aim of the Maudsley NDU has been to develop bridging therapy, a new approach to nursing care aimed at bridging the gap between hospital and community; this improves care delivery and promotes community integration for those with acute mental health problems. Bridging therapy is based on the principle of continuing care and utilises, (a) the developed nurse-patient relationship, and (b) the flexibility of the therapeutic plan to be implemented where necessary. The gap is bridged by extending the role of the primary nurse to support the client after discharge. Six stages are involved: admission; assessment of post-discharge needs; establishment of post-discharge plans; discharge; intensive monitoring of bridging therapy; reduced support of bridging therapy; termination. This work is being evaluated to explore clinical outcomes and cost implications. (Maudsley NDU Bridging Therapy 1994, Rainsford and Caan 1994)

Poverty and health needs

The area in which Strelley NDU is based is one where there is considerable poverty and deprivation with an average Jarman score of around + 45. A scheme was developed to assess the impact of health visiting on the health needs associated with poverty. The main purpose behind this work was to develop a model of health-visiting practice which was responsive to local need rather than following traditional medical/child-health surveillance programmes, and which could be transferred to other areas of deprivation.

A second strand to this work has been the development of a partnership approach when working with families. This brings to light some of the invisible long-term work which is undertaken with families in deprived settings. Case studies spanning time have been used to demonstrate both short-term goals (e.g. immunisation) and longer-term goals such as child or parent safety. (see Boyd *et al.* 1995; Periton and Perkins, 1995)

Use of dementia care mapping

Dementia care mapping is primarily a method for developmental evaluation of care. It not only provides an audit of quality of interpersonal care and well-being of people with dementia, but also potential for growth and change.

One of the wards in Seacroft (wards V and W) NDU has supported four members of staff to undertake the basic course in dementia care mapping over the last two years, two of whom have gone on to complete the advanced course. (All courses are facilitated by the Bradford Dementia Research Group). The ward has demonstrated that using dementia care mapping in 1994 and 1995 has provided a significant improvement in the quality of care. Workshops and discussions have been held for ward staff; there have been dissemination workshops in the NDU for staff within the trust and outside, and much of the discussions have focused on the philosophy underpinning dementia care mapping. The four qualified users of dementia care mapping are regularly asked to help carry out evaluative work on other wards within the trust and they have also been asked to assist in the use of dementia care mapping as a research instrument on another ward within the trust. (Seacroft (wards V and W) NDU Second Annual Report)

The SARA project

Homefield Place NDU at Seaford has been developing individual activity programmes for the patients. Activity was established using dementia care mapping and this led to the development and implementation of the Social and Recreational Assessment form (SARA) into care planning. In this way an opportunity was developed for patients to continue with their normal leisure activities such as watching a favourite television programme, singing in the choir or listening to the music they enjoy. A nursing assistant post has been re-profiled as a social and recreational assistant to work under the guidance of the primary nurse and to help fulfil the client's social and recreational needs. An audit of the associated standard indicated that 60% of clients had completed SARAs and the information was incorporated into their care plans. (Homefield Place NDU Review 1993–1994)

Health education packages

Health education has become a nursing function in the West Dorset NDU. Primary nurses have identified a key role in improving information and in the provision of advice on health and disease-related issues. Under the direction of one primary nurse, health education packages were developed relating to a number of medical conditions on the unit. Ranging from heart disease/disorders, asthma and diabetes to gastro-intestinal disorders, the packages contain useful published information, as well as leaflets devised by nurses interested in a particular topic. Monthly displays on health matters are also used.

See also page 67

Medication education

The introduction of programmes which help people continue with or learn to take responsibility for their own medications has been widespread in the NDUs. It was the starting point of work for Truth NDU and has been one of the major areas of work for Glenfield as part of the realisation of their philosophy of self-care.

See also page 58

Another example is at Seacroft (wards V and W) NDU where, having noted the disempowering effects of the removal of patients' medication on admission, the team concluded that a medication education programme should be opened. This involved changing procedures regarding details collected on admission and during the 72-hour assessment period. Instead, they developed a package that will enable nurses to assess patients' knowledge of their medication on admission, during the assessment and again before discharge. This was achieved by conducting a literature review on self-medication, attending a study day and conference, visiting another ward with the regime and asking the advice of the pharmacist. The long-term goal is for self-medication' which is particularly challenging for this client group of elderly mentally-infirm people. (Seacroft (wards V and W) Second Annual Report)

Carers emergency alert card

Following an incident where a carer collapsed leaving his dependent relative uncared for, Homefield Place NDU have devised a card which is carried by the carer of a dependent person. The information is held centrally on an index file, and if the carer has an accident and the dependent person is potentially left in a vulnerable position alone, the staff of the unit will respond and assist by arranging support services.

Carers have confirmed, by evaluation, that this provides them with 24-hour support and peace of mind. Following two years of active use in Seaford, the scheme has been expanded county-wide. In a multi-agency project, the community trust, the social services department and Care for the Carers have developed the scheme and through the county telephone LifeLine service run by the district councils, it is available to a potential 5000 carers. (Phair 1995)

Organisation of Care

The way in which care is organised and delivered is clearly fundamental to the running of the units. Some of the endeavours have, as their main aim, the improved continuity of care for patients and clients. Others focus on access to services, and a number are quite clearly initiatives for assuring the quality of the service provided. Examples have been included in this section that relate to new patterns of service provision.

Continuity of care

The first examples in this section relate to ways in which units have sought to improve continuity of care which has been linked to endeavours that go beyond the confines of the NDU and impinge on organisational changes. Some have been driven by policy initiatives such as Changing Childbirth (DoH 1992) while others have been developed in response to local need.

Providing continuity of care and choice

The aim in the Wistow Midwifery NDU has been the integration of community and hospital midwifery teams to create a seamless service that provides continuity of care. This has required role expansion (e.g. hospital-based midwives working in the community and vice versa); greater autonomy for managing the low-risk caseload; and universal client-held records throughout the period of care. The work has had major organisational as well as clinical implications and has taken a long time to establish. Attention has been given not only to skill development but to the changes required in such things as shift patterns, travel and transport, and team structures, taking into account the personal and family needs of the midwives as well as those of the organisation. After much effort and change the team are now able to demonstrate a model of care delivery in line with the recommendations of *Changing Childbirth* and are working towards pre-defined targets in relation to continuity of care and choice within a group practice model. (Walsh 1995)

Continuity of care and care management

Andover NDU has established a system of continuity of care where district nurses retain responsibility for care planning should any patients require admission to the community hospital. This is linked with a unit project for training the district nurse as a care manager. A pilot project has been jointly funded with social services and there have been demonstrations of the effectiveness and benefits of having a care manager who is a district nurse. While complex problems had to be solved so that the district nurse could maintain responsibility for inpatient care, ways have been sought to establish good working relations in the team. The district nurse also has access to community care money via social services. Following patient assessment, the district nurse can plan and implement nursing and social care and evaluate that care throughout the patient's need for services. (Andover NDU 1994)

Case management

Newcastle NDU has concentrated primarily on the introduction of case management. This involves a case manager (a nurse) being appointed for a particular group of patients, who is responsible for the 'path of managed care', that is the predicted progress expected for patients with similar clinical problems throughout their stay in hospital, from admission to discharge. Controlling the standards of quality and cost of patient care are key elements of case management, as are establishing the desired outcomes and the services and resources needed to achieve them. Collaborative planning plays an important part within the multi-disciplinary team to ensure a co-ordinated and organised approach.

The programme is outlined in diagnostic related group (DRG) care maps and it is the case manager's responsibility to record an individual's progress along the pathway, dealing with any variations as they arise. The work has spanned four areas: the development of the managed care system; development of a research design for evaluation; choosing a model of case management to be implemented; and education of case managers.

The model chosen for use in this unit involved an extension of the primary nurse role to include case management activities. Education has been provided in collaboration with a local university and college of health studies, and has included a programme for case managers and a course on advanced nursing practice dealing mainly with case management and managed care.

Links have also been made with the USA where this approach was developed, and visits made by members of the team. Similarly, visitors from the USA have been to the unit and supported the initiative. The experience of case management and care maps has been disseminated within the trusts, and they are being introduced in other specialities. (Hale 1995, Laxade and Hale 1995, Royal Victoria Hospital NDU, Newcastle 1994)

Access to services

A difficulty which many places experience is a ready access to services which is acceptable to both patients and staff; in this way attention can be given quickly to needs, waiting-times can be reduced and the range and number of services can be increased. Below are different methods employed by NDUs to deal with this issue.

Admissions and work schedules

The team at Weston Park NDU was concerned that centrally-controlled patient admissions often led to prolonged waits before they could be attended to. A member of the team has been an active contributor to the trust-wide SIGMA project, supported by Trent Region, which led to ward managers controlling admission to allow for individual attention.

To respond to the changes of admission patterns nurses started to work flexible schedules. Initially this meant that a nurse would begin a shift an hour or two later than usual and would finish later. This was the subject of a full investigation by a work psychologist to evaluate the impact of change in work schedules on the performance and well-being of staff. (see Smith 1995)

Increased referrals

As a result of their development work East Berkshire NDU was able to accept a significant increase in the number of new referrals of patients with severe behavioural problems. This was in part due to the personal relationships group work undertaken by two team-members which led to better systems of contact and communication. Considerable effort went into forging good interpersonal relations between the behavioural support team and other members of the trust, as well as ensuring that others were fully aware of the skills of the team and ways in which the service could be used. Referrals continued to increase through 1995. A waiting list has been established which led the team to develop priorities for referrals but also confirms the value of the service they provide. (East Berkshire NDU 1995)

Use of situational analysis to explore future options

Byron NDU has used situational analysis to provide an overview of the present and future business environment through demand and demand trends. The framework they have adopted is Cohen (1987) which examines four environs – situation (including demands and trends for the product by the customers targeted); neutral (financial and legislative elements); competitor (competing elements); and company (the situation within the unit, including resources and strengths and weaknesses). By assessing the current situation of the unit in relation its working environment they can plan the services they will offer in the light of wider circumstances. (Byron Ward Business Report 1995)

Quality initiatives

A major aim of all NDUs is to improve the quality of service they offer to patients and clients. Thus quality initiatives are related to many aspects of their work. The examples included in this section demonstrate some of the ways this has been addressed by the units.

Implementing protocols

See also page 23

Although Liverpool NDU has used the clinical fellowship scheme as a developmental process for staff this work has also had a marked impact on practice. Early implementation of the protocols helped to highlight staff knowledge gaps, leading to needs-driven educational programmes. It has also highlighted the difference in levels of clinical competence between newly qualified and more experienced staff with implications for skill-mix and staff-development opportunities.

The core protocols act as bench marks for good practice both within and beyond the NDU. They have helped to make nursing care more visible and can be used as a means of ensuring best practice. Most importantly, feedback from patients indicates a high degree of involvement and satisfaction leading, as one patient said, to 'more control of my own care.' (see Waterworth and Byrne 1995, Boon 1994)

Quality initiatives

Part of the work of Cartmel NDU has been a standard-setting project. A number of standards have been generated using the Lakeview model (McFadden and Gadd 1995), which have included client involvement through community meetings. The standards are under the ownership and control of the clients and clinical team, and peer audit ensures that they are monitored regularly and maintained. Core standards have been implemented in response to purchaser requirements, and a recent independent audit has shown that ten out of twelve are being met.

As part of quality assurance Qualpacs (Wandelt 1975) study sessions were set up on the West Dorset NDU with the help of an external expert. Subsequent audits have identified that some of the work being undertaken by nurses was not appropriate to their skills but would be better undertaken by a ward housekeeper and a ward co-ordinator. These two new positions have now been created within the ward team and people are in post. Whilst the use of Qualpacs has been useful, some difficulties have been experienced implementing it owing to the need to release staff from the ward for both training and assessing. Discussions have been held with the trust's audit department to take this forward.

NDUs are committed to a quality service and Weston Park Hospital NDU helps to ensure this by the use of quality cycles through a three-staged process. Stage one is the measurement of observed nursing practice. Stage two is the comparison of practice with expectations, involving standard setting. The third stage is the implementation of change to reconcile discrepancies between observations and expectations. The ward now has many standards which have been developed following a protocol involving both exploration of the literature and drawing on the experience of other units. In each instance the standards have defined anticipated outcomes against which they can assess their own progress. All the ward staff have attended teaching sessions regarding what standards are, how they are set, how they are audited and ways in which action plans can be formed to tackle problems. Areas considered include, amongst others, the named nurse concept; admission to the ward; discharge from the ward and pressure area assessment. (see Logan 1993)

Computerised care-based protocols

East Berkshire NDU has been developing research-based care protocols. These will be incorporated into a computerised client information system (CIS) in order to explore the impact of processes of care on outcomes. This project has demonstrated the challenges of working with external consultants. Despite promising initial discussions with one company the outcome was disappointing. For example, it did not include all aspects of assessment, and was too expensive, which led to delay. The NDU's computerisation of client assessments and consumer information is now being integrated with the trust's information management system (CIMS) which will ultimately lead to a package that will integrate more readily with other trust systems. Training and continued implementation of the system continued until mid-1996. The information should help produce data on the client's quality of life. (East Berkshire NDU 1995)

Information technology

The long-term objectives for the Cartmel NDU IT project have comprised the evaluation and possible adoption of resource management, nursing information systems and computerised care planning. Initially, the most important aim was to help nursing staff become computer literate and feel comfortable working with new technology. Towards the end of the second year of the project, nursing staff completed a questionnaire to measure their knowledge levels and to assess their views on how it was progressing. The responses indicated a greater understanding of information technology and computers and a greater confidence and willingness to try new ideas. A number of benefits identified by staff included: speedy access to information; the saving of time; professionally produced reports and information packages; the learning of new skills; easier monitoring of information; more effective channels of communication. A number of obstacles were also identified: lack of formal training; too much time away from the clinical area; lack of confidence; lack of support from other agencies within the hospital; on the whole, however, these were far outweighed by the benefits.

Cartmel has since been instrumental in accessing the Internet and established their own conferences, workshops and international dialogues. They have noted the scarcity of material related to nursing practice and have made five information booklets prepared by the unit available through the Internet as well as publishing them in hard copy. (see Gadd 1995)

Audit of nursing time and skill mix

In order to explore skill mix, Homefield Place NDU at Seaford carried out an audit of nursing time. This told them that in one week the nurses spent 36 hours on non-nursing duties including laundry, washing up, car maintenance and administrative and clerical work. After discussion with other departments and allocating tasks elsewhere this inappropriate use of time has now been halved. It was further reduced by the introduction of a part-time ward clerk. In addition, an audit was carried out of nurse-client contact time and it was found that staff spent at most four hours with a client each week. By introducing different methods it became possible to increase this to 12 hours per client. Primary nursing was recommended as the most efficient way of effecting this change. (Phair 1993).

Developing Roles

The development of nursing and support roles has been of supreme importance in many of units. This has achieved by expanding existing roles, establishing new ones and spending time in role development through both formal educational processes and supervisory means.

Expanding current roles

Role expansion, in this context, is taken as meaning the way in which members of the clinical team have widened the range of services which they are able to offer patients either through developing new skills or accepting additional responsibility for a different range of work. There has been much talk of role extension, commonly understood as the learning of a new, often technical, skill. However, role expansion focuses much more strongly on recognition of gaps in services for patients and clients and developing ways to meet those needs. It may, or may not, include learning new technical skills but this aspect of the development is the means to role expansion rather than an end in its own right.

Role expansion

Role expansion is a common phenomenon within the NDUs. For example, nurses throughout Glenfield NDU have developed and expanded their role since publication of the Scope of Professional Practice (1992). This has been helped by the development of clinical skills such as phlebotomy, cannulation, removal of femoral arterial sheaths, and administering IV cardiac drugs. (*Nursing Standard News* 1994). One of the team members has moved on to run the recently opened day-care unit for cardiology patients which is a nurse-led service. Other areas which may develop in the future are greater involvement with the out-patient department and nurse-led clinics.

The role of nurse practitioner at Annex NDU is one where the clinical skills of RMNs has been developed to an advanced level. All staff are engaged on personal development programmes and further training to enable them to function autonomously and provide a multi-skilled service to patients. The nurse practitioner role is being examined by an external consultant (Lathlean 1996)

In the Worthing NDU nursing roles have been expanded to facilitate nurse-led treatments. This was stimulated by a concern that many patients who required cytotoxic treatments had to travel thirty miles to a specialist centre as the service was not available locally. The few patients treated locally experienced long waiting times until junior doctors, who where busy on the wards, could attend the day-care unit. In addition, these doctors were inexperienced in accessing difficult veins and administering drugs. In close collaboration with the consultant, over the past five years the nurses have taken over total management of the day ward and are now responsible not only for administration of the cytotoxic treatments but also for a range of other services such as family support groups, phone-in helplines, management of side effects of treatment and a lymphoedema service. The number of patients seen in the unit has increased three-fold in this time as has the range of conditions which can be managed locally. A computerised record-keeping system has been introduced and some of these data are being studied as part of a programme of evaluation. (Sitzia and Dikken 1996)

Introducing new roles

Another approach has been the introduction of new roles in response to local needs. In some instances the whole team has been involved in exploring ways in which a new role can be integrated within an already established service which has led to adjustments in the way the team functions. Thus the work goes beyond the description and development of the role itself and highlights the wider need to consider how the incumbent will function within the team as an organic whole.

Public health project

Stepney NDU, based in an area of high deprivation, established the Public Health Project which was started with the belief that the success of health promotion work, aimed at changes in the life choices of individuals, depends not only on a healthy environment but must also acknowledge the structural constraints placed on these choices. The aims of the project were:

- to define the empowerment work done by community nurses and to press for this to be recognised and purchased as Public Health Nursing
- to develop ways to overcome the existing structural constraints affecting on the health of clients individually and collectively
- to identify key public health issues for community nurses and health-care users
- to develop new structures within nursing that will provide the environmental context necessary for health gain

The project works through a multi-agency group and their respective networks. Housing has been the focus of attention and achievements include:

- joint working with a local firm of solicitors to develop training in housing issues for health workers and acting as a practical resource for clients
- a workshop and seminar for staff to identify the most common housing problems that clients said affected their health
- a collaborative primary health-care based housing clinic
- a joint NDU/King's Fund workshop with purchasers and providers in three agencies (housing, health and social services) and two London boroughs
- seeking funding for the regeneration of one especially deprived area, the Ocean Estate
- setting up a fuel, poverty and home energy efficiency health promotion project

This has been a change from the more traditional way in which the team functioned, shifting towards a wider multi-agency approach and giving many members the opportunity to develop projects of their own related to the needs of the local population. (see Stepney NDU Annual Report 1994, Buxton and Savigar 1993)

Introduction of public health role

Strelley NDU (Health Visiting) introduced the role of the health visitor, public health, to work with local people and explore their needs; to co-ordinate and develop ways to respond to those needs and translate Health of the Nation Targets into action; and to work with others to bring about improvements to the immediate environment and increase local resources for health. Introduction of this role was partly stimulated by multi-agency working and partly by a need to prioritise resources. More importantly it was felt that the services offered should match local needs if the health and welfare of the population with whom they worked was to be influenced. This has led to specific projects such as accident prevention, multi-agency work, management of smoking and solvent abuse, and women's health.

Accident prevention was directed at the under fives because of high morbidity in this group. The intention has been to raise public awareness of the causes of accidents and how to apply first aid measures. This consisted of supplying safety equipment, teaching first aid, and discussing with families ways of providing a safe home. There was also multi-agency work with housing and transport departments which has received a high level of local support.

Initiatives in respect of smoking cessation and solvent abuse have included training for health and community workers, the promotion of support groups, and education opportunities for users.

Local women had also mentioned problems with isolation, loneliness and poor mental health, which were confirmed by information from case-load profiles. Consequently, a leisure group was established by local people, supported by the health visitors, to participate in leisure and health activities. In addition, a women's aid counselling session was set up in response to an increasing awareness of the levels of violence experienced by local women. Similarly a women's forum for workers concerned with domestic violence was established to aid communication and provide mutual support between workers, an initiative supported by the health-visiting team.

Information about the work which this team have undertaken in the introduction of public health to health visiting has been widely disseminated and is now being replicated in other areas. (see Boyd *et al.* 1993; Brummell and Perkins 1995)

Development of emergency nurse practitioner programme

Dewsbury NDU has developed the role of the accident and emergency nurse into that of an Emergency Nurse Practitioner (ENP). This began with an information-gathering exercise both within and outside the unit. Arising from the belief that preparation should be practice driven, an awayday was held to seek the views of the unit team about the scope of the ENP and the learning requirements. As a result of this, an ENP programme (pathway) has been prepared. The pathway comprises ten modules which have been accredited by the local university and delivered by the unit in partnership with the college of health, namely: research awareness; advanced anatomy and physiology; assessment; casting; venous access and administration of IV medication; intubation; nurse prescribing; management of ventricular fibrillation; choice modules and action research. At a time of rapid growth in the work of nurses in accident and emergency departments, particularly in their autonomous role in managing minor injuries, this work is of particular relevance to the safeguarding of standards and assurance of competence. (Bland 1996)

Development of non-nurse ward co-ordinator role

Ashington (ward 5) NDU has been developing a non-nurse ward co-ordinator role. The traditional nurse-in-charge system, where one qualified nurse takes responsibility for co-ordinating ward activities on each shift is difficult to reconcile with a caseload approach. The nurse in charge is usually also a primary or associate nurse and therefore experiences the demand of performing two conflicting roles at once. The role of the non-nurse ward co-ordinator is an attempt to address this problem by using non-qualified personnel with the right skills and abilities to co-ordinate general ward activities. This takes the burden of general administrative and clerical tasks off qualified nurses, allowing them to concentrate on their clinical role. It also allows senior nurses to develop an effective staff development and support role, since their time and energy is not being sapped by routine administrative and clerical tasks. Ashington NDU has found it tremendously successful both in improving the nursing service to patients and in increasing general ward efficiency. (see Kay 1993)

Introducing maternity support workers

Ensuring continuity of care has been an important aim for the midwives in Bournemouth NDU. This is not always easy to achieve however when, for example, women develop difficulties in labour and require transfer to the obstetric unit in Poole. Following a visit to Holland, the midwives have taken the idea of the Kraam Verzorgsteren (lying-in helpers) and adapted this approach to meet their local needs. A 12-week programme has been developed taking into account both theoretical and practical learning, the content of which is matched to the job description of the Maternity Support Worker. It is anticipated that by introducing this role, which deals with some of the housekeeping and clerical work as well as offering basic support to mothers with supervision from the midwives, the midwives themselves will be able to spend more time providing a direct service for mothers. (Husbands and Hall 1996)

Redefining roles and responsibilities

In some instances more traditional roles have been developed, not only to increase the job satisfaction of the incumbents but also in order that clinical expertise can be developed further. In this way best use can be made of clinical skills to ensure that patients and clients receive optimal care.
In some cases the initiative has concerned whole teams and in others the development has focused on individual team members but in both cases it has brought advantages to both the participants and the patients.

Redefining primary nursing roles

Liverpool NDU had been undertaking primary nursing for a while but felt that the time had come to reconsider and fine tune the way in which care was managed. Their concerns focused around ensuring that there was opportunity for continuing development of both primary nurses and associate nurses who had gained considerable experience in their current roles. After much debate they introduced the role of care co-ordinator, a senior experienced primary nurse who would lead a team of less experienced nurses, help them to gain the skills of primary nursing under supervision and manage the team, as well as providing care for an agreed number of patients; this has given them the change to enhance their managerial role while still making best use of their clinical expertise. It has also provided developmental opportunities for more junior members in a relatively stable team, affording them new learning opportunities and expanding their skills and knowledge of clinical care within a safe environment. (Waterworth 1996)

Seacroft (wards V and W) NDU is also expanding the primary nursing role. Their particular concern has been proper management of the discharge of their clients, many of whom are highly dependant. To this end they are developing Outreach Primary Nursing as a means of ensuring that the links between home and hospital are strengthened and there is integration between the two areas when considering care needs. (Gordon 1993, Gordon 1995)

Development of local experts

Like many of the other units Andover NDU has developed local 'experts' who offer a range of services including, for example, the diabetic liaison nurse, stoma care clinic, carers group, and the cancer support group. These people can be called upon by colleagues to give advice and support and, in some instances, take over care management. In this way a wider use of knowledge-based practice can be assured, thus increasing the quality of the service offered to patients. (Andover NDU 1994)

This development is mirrored in many of the other units. For example, wound care has become the specialist area of expertise for a member of the Homeward team in Brighton (Phelan *et al.* 1992), nutrition has been focused on in Southport NDU (McQuire 1992) and specialist investigations in Glenfield NDU. (Glenfield NDU 1995)

Primary nurse development programme

Truth Ward NDU has implemented a system of primary nursing alongside a primary nurse development programme. Primary nursing has been audited and the following are examples of resulting initiatives:

- redefinition of the roles of primary and associate nurses and the role of health-care support workers
- creating a primary nurse development programme
- redesigning a patients' and relatives' information booklet
- the decision to allow D grade nurses to take on the role of a primary nurse with support

The programme aims to ensure that all primary nurses are familiar with their roles and have a good understanding of the wider issues related to them. It also offers participants guidance to reach the full potential of their role as advanced practitioners. (Mills 1995)

A primary nursing development programme has also been developed in Glenfield NDU as part of their policy of supporting self-care in the unit. In preparation for this, work was undertaken to clarify a shared understanding of primary nursing and its use in practice. The programme itself is also being evaluated as part of a wider strategy. (Furlong 1994, 1995, 1996)

See also page 126

Developing SHO training

Royal Bournemouth Hospital NDU has identified the need for the training of medical staff (senior house officers) in relation to the service provided by the unit, to ensure that they become familiar with low-risk obstetric care as well as the more complex technical needs of women in high-risk groups. This was agreed with the obstetric consultants. A package has been developed which includes an introduction to the philosophy of the unit, the criteria for delivery in the unit and the training programme. In this it is clearly stated that the SHO will work with a midwife for one day each week for eight weeks. The programme includes ante natal, intra partum and post-natal care in the maternity unit and time with a community midwife. Participants are also invited to join the parent craft and relaxation classes. As the majority of SHOs in the hospital are going to be GPs, it is felt that this should give them valuable insight into the work of the midwife and normal maternity care. (see Thomas 1994)

Cascade model of clinical supervision

Clinical supervision is common to the NDUs but the way in which each unit is tackling it varies. For example, Liverpool NDU has developed a cascade model with the ward manager as the lynch pin. It is not a hierarchical management model, but a means of generating a network of support and development for the whole team. It also offers the opportunity for less experienced members to develop this aspect of their role to enhance their own development and prepare them for a wider range of responsibilities. A role evaluation instrument has been produced and this is to be reviewed internally and externally. An educational programme has also been developed as an adjunct. The detailed framework and the educational programme are presented in Waterworth (1995b).

Trajectory project

Oxford 7E NDU noted that despite one of the lowest sickness/absence levels in the hospital, the staff turnover rate was above average in 1994. To explore why, and to examine the patterns and trends of staff departure, a trajectory project was undertaken. Findings indicated that the NDU had operated for some time as a breeding ground for the profession, with 31% of the 35 staff leaving for promotion and 21% to undertake further education. Six were promotions to posts outside the trust, including four of the most senior staff. The trajectory concluded that whilst staff turnover was higher than desirable for the trust, the profession at large benefited. (Northcott 1995)

SUMMARY

Development work is the bread and butter of NDU activities where, when a gap in services is identified, the team ensure that action is taken to fill that need. All the units have used a range of development activities, many of which are primarily concerned with giving more control to patients and clients. For example, the majority of in-patient services are using self-medication programmes (e.g. Glenfield), bedside handover is common practice (e.g. Southport, Bowthorpe) and patient or client-held records are widely used. In essence, simple those these practices may sound, they do indicate a fundamental shift from the traditional model of control by health professionals to a shared model of equality.

However, it can be seen that development work of this nature takes time. A common experience shared by many of the units has been that their original plans were rather over-ambitious and the amount of time which was needed to change practice was greater than they had anticipated. Similarly, some had not foreseen some of the obstacles they would have to face in order to introduce new services or change old ways, particularly when it was necessary to negotiate beyond the confines of the unit itself which has been the case in most of the work undertaken. Helping nurses to think strategically in order to see beyond these confines and plan in both the short and the long term has been an essential lesson arising from this work. Some of these experiences, including indications of what did and what did not work, have been explored as a central theme in order that they can be shared with others. (Marsh and MacAlpine 1996)

Critical lessons have also been learned which relate to ensuring that the right person is doing the right job rather than fiercely guarding boundaries. For example, while some of the new roles which have been developed have offered opportunities for nurses and midwives to expand their work, this has meant that they have also had to develop skills and accept responsibility for areas of work previously undertaken by others. From time to time this has raised debate about whether the work they are doing is truly nursing. However, if the service is viewed from the perspective of the patient or client who requires a comprehensive care-giver rather than being passed from one person to another because of the focus of traditional boundaries of responsibility then this argument can readily be disputed. In the same light, some of the new roles have been concerned with the introduction of new team members such as interpreters, or clerical and support staff requiring different use of the same resources; this is a potential reduction in the number of nursing staff employed. However it is neither good use of time for clinical staff to undertake work which could be done by people without the requisite professional quali-fication nor does it lead to job satisfaction when those concerned are diverted from clini-cal care. Thus these adjustments have proved to be of value.

It is gratifying to see that many of the areas in which development has taken place are common to many of the units since this helps to identify the common focus of work which helps to improve patient and client care. Developing local experts in any area will assist in ensuring the use of knowledge-based practice; steps to return control to patients such as self-medication and patient education will support users in becoming more empowered to manage their own health; developing new skills which are specific to a clinical speciality will help to increase the range of choice and continuity of care; and exploring ways in which roles can be developed will enhance both job satisfaction and the quality of patient care. Lessons can be learned not only from units with a similar clinical interest but in a wide range of specialities, all of which highlight the shared expertise of nursing practice.

References & related reading

Adair E (1994) 'The patients' agenda – what do patients really think about the care they receive in hospital?' *Nursing Standard* 9(9) 20–23

Adair E (1996) *An investigation of the use of story-telling interviews with discharged patients as a method of generating quality improvement initiatives* 7E NDU Oxford, Radcliffe Hospital

Andover NDU *Annual Report* (1994)

Anston Ward NDU (1993–4) *Annual Report* Rampton Hospital

Bland A (1996) 'Developing the role of the emergency nurse practitioner: the approach taken by a nursing development unit' *European Nurse* Vol 1 no 2

Boon A (1994) *The Need For Clinical Supervision* Royal Liverpool and Broadgreen University NHS Trust

Boyd M, Brummell K, Billingham K, Perkins E (1993) *The Public Health Post at Strelley: an interim report* Nottingham Community Health NHS Trust, Strelley NDU

Boyd M, Marley L, Perkins E (1995) *Poverty and Health Needs: How Can Health Visiting Respond?* Nottingham Community Health NHS Trust, Strelley NDU

Brummell K, Perkins E (1995) *Public Health at Strelley: A Model in Action* Nottingham Community Health NHS Trust, Strelley NDU

Buxton V (1993) 'A healthy start in life' *Nursing Standard* 8(10) 18–20

Buxton V, Savigar S (1993) 'Public Health Nursing – Grasping the Nettle' *Primary Health Care* 3(5)

Byron Ward NDU *Business Report* (1995) King's Healthcare

Chadwick D (1996) *Bedside Handover: giving patients the lead in their care* Norfolk and Norwich Healthcare NHS Trust, Bowthorpe NDU

Chadwick D, Mitchell K (1996) *Self Medication: helping patients to remain independent* Norfolk and Norwich Healthcare NHS Trust, Bowthorpe NDU

Chelsea and Westminster Intensive Care and NDU *Annual Report* July 1994–June 1995

Clarke M, Sheppard B (1992) 'From Patient to Person: A Patient's Forum' in Black G *Nursing Development Units Work in Progress* London, King's Fund

Cohen (1994) 'Food For Thought' *Health Services Journal* Apr 7 104(5397) 12

Cohen W (1987) *Developing a Winning Market Plan* Winchester, John Wiley

Copperman J, Morrison P (1995) *We Thought We Knew: Involving Patients in Nursing Practice* London, King's Fund

Department of Health (1993) *Changing Childbirth: report of the expert maternity group* London, HMSO

Denison A (1994) *The Named Nurse Concept.* Internal Report. Sheffield, Weston Park NDU

Dodd T (1994) 'Clients' art and ethics' *Nursing Times* 90(11) 24

Dodd T (1994) 'Developing Mental Health Nursing', *Nursing Developments News* December, London, King's Fund

Dunford M (1995) 'Responding to need' *Nursing Developments News* 11 (June) 3–4 London, King's Fund

Dutton J M, Grylls L, Goldstone L A (1991) *Accident and Emergency Nursing Monitor: an audit of the quality of nursing care in hospital accident and emergency departments* Gale Centre Publications

East Berkshire NDU *Annual Report* October 1994–September 1995

East Berkshire NHS Trust Behavioural Support Team (1996) *Developing Best Practice*

Evans A, Griffiths P (1994) *The Development of a Nursing-led In-patient Service* London, King's Fund

Fascione J (1995) 'Healing Power of Touch' *Elderly Care* 7(1) 19–21

Furlong S (1994) 'Primary Nursing: a new philosophy' *British Journal of Nursing* 3(13) 668–671

Furlong S (1995a) 'Self Care: the application of a ward philosophy' *Journal of Clinical Nursing* 5(2) 85–90

Furlong S (1995b) *Self Care: Application in Practice* London, King's Fund

Furlong S (1995c) 'An Observation of the roles of primary and associate nurses in practice' *British Journal of Nursing* in press

Furlong S (1995d) 'Primary Nursing: nurses' perceptions of what enhances and what diminishes its success in practice' *British Journal of Nursing* in press

Furlong S (1996) 'Do self-administration of medicines programmes enhance patient knowledge, compliance and satisfaction?' *Journal of Advanced Nursing* 23(6) 1254–62

Gadd D (1995) *Information Technology* Cartmel NDU, Mental Health Services of Salford NHS Trust

Gadd D, Mahood N (1995) *Clinical Supervision: a time for professional development* Cartmel NDU, Mental Health Services of Salford NHS Trust

Gilley J, David N (1995) 'The living room' *Elderly Care Journal* 7(3) 9–12

Glasper E A, Lowson S Manger R, Phillips L (1995) 'Developing a centre for health information and promotion' *British Journal of Nursing* 4(12) 693–697

Glenfield NDU *The Past Three Years* 1992–5

Goddard N (1996) *Turning ideas into reality: the patient information pack – information for all* Norfolk and Norwich Healthcare NHS Trust, Bowthorpe NDU

Gordon A (1995) 'Revolving door system' *Elderly Care* 7(4) 9–12

Gordon A (1993) *Outreach Primary Nursing* Seacroft (wards V and W) NDU, Seacroft Leeds

Hale C (1995) 'Research issues in case management' *Nursing Standard* 9(44) 29–32

Halek C, Cremin D, Chandran U, Parnell J (1995) 'Weight on their minds' *Nursing Times* 91(48) 42–43

Halek C (1994) 'The weigh forward' *Nursing Management* 11(2) 6–7

Holly C (1996) 'Focus on Need' *Nursing Times* 92(3) 46–47

Horner J (1992) 'A Carers' Panel: enabling relatives to influence patient care' in Black G *Nursing Developments Work in Progress* London, King's Fund

Husbands S, Thomas M (1994) *Setting up a midwifery-led Unit* Royal Bournemouth Maternity Unit, Bournemouth and Christchurch Hospital NHS Trust

Husbands S, Hall S M, (1996) *Maternity Support Worker Project* Royal Bournemouth Maternity Unit, Bournemouth and Christchurch Hospital NHS Trust

James J (1995) 'Children speak out about health' *Primary Health Care* 5(10)

Kay J (1993) 'Sharing the Burden' *Nursing Times* 89(36) 34–36

Lathlean J (1996) *The Role of the Nurse Practitioner in Annex NDU: the findings of an interview study* Annex NDU, Pathfinder Trust

Laxade S, Hale C (1995) 'Managed Care 2: an opportunity for nursing' *British Journal of Nursing* 14 6 345–350

Littlewood S, Saeidi S (1994) 'Therapeutic Mealtimes' *Elderly Care* 6(6) 20–21

Logan R (1993) *Standard Setting and Audit* Internal Report, Weston Park NDU, Sheffield.

Lowson S (1995) 'The growth of an NDU in a paediatric out-patient department' *British Journal of Nursing* 4(1) 36–38

Marsh S, MacAlpine M (1996) *Our Own Capabilities – clinical nurse managers taking a strategic approach to service improvement* London, King's Fund

Maudsley NDU 'Bridging Therapy' *Annual Report* December 1993–November 1994

McFadden K, Gadd D (1995) *Quality Initiatives: Emphasising Client Involvement in the Nursing Process* Cartmel NDU, Mental Health Services of Salford NHS Trust

McQuire (1992) 'Promoting nutritional awareness: opportunities provided by a hospital stay' in Black G *Nursing Developments Work in Progress* London, King's Fund

Mills C (1995) 'Transfer to the ward from ICU: families' experiences' *Nursing in Critical Care* Pilot Edition 22–24

Mills C (1995) 'Evaluation of primary nursing in a nursing development unit' *Nursing Times* 91(39) 34–37

Morrison P (1992) 'Challenges for clinical leaders' *Nursing Developments News* 1, Dec 5

Morton S (1995) 'Nurse 95 Awards' *Nursing Standard* 6(12) 53

Northcott N (1996) 'The significance of culture in an NDU' *Nursing Developments News* 15 (June) 3–5

Northcott N (1995) *Career Trajectories for Nurses Working in NDU* Internal Report 7E NDU Oxford, Radcliffe Hospital

Nursing Standard (1992) news report 6(40), no 40 p16

Nursing Standard (1994) 'It's A family Affair' 8(34) 20–22

Orem D (1991) *Nursing: Concepts of Practice* 4th edition, New York, MacGraw Hill

Oxford Radcliffe Hospital NDU Annual Report (1995–6) *The Place of Complementary Therapies in Nursing*

Periton C, Perkins E (1995) *Working in Partnership: Health Visiting in an Area of Deprivation* Strelley NDU Nottingham Community Health NHS Trust

Phair L (1993) *An Audit of Nursing Time and Activity* unpublished, internal report, Seaford NDU

Phair L (1995) 'A card to give carers more peace of mind' *Nursing Standard* 91(34) 24–25

Phelan P, Hawkey B, Sheppard B (1992) 'Wound Management: research alongside care' in Black G *Nursing Developments Work in Progress* London, King's Fund

Phillips L (1995) 'Enuresis in children' in *Nursing Times* vol 91, no 42 p64

Rainsford E, Caan W (1994) 'Experience of supervising discharges' *Journal Of Clinical Nursing* 3(3) 133–137

Rees J (1995) *A Taste of your Medication* unpublished MSc dissertation, University of Northumbria

Royal Bournemouth Hospital NDU *Maternity Unit Report* 1996

Royal Liverpool and Broadgreen University Trust NDU, *Final Report* 1995

Royal Victoria Infirmary NDU *Annual Report* 1993–4

Seacroft (wards Vand W) Hospital NDU, *Second Annual Report* 1994

Sheehan A (1994) 'Extending the role of mental health nurses' *Nursing Standard* 8(44) 31–34

Sheffield Occupational Health NDU *Annual Report* 1993–4 Sheffield City Council

Sheffield Occupational Health NDU *Annual Report* 1994–5 Sheffield City Council

Shephard J and Garbett R (1993) 'A question of choice' *Nursing Times* Vol 29 no 12 50–52

Sheppard B (1994) *Looking Back – Moving Forward: Developing Elderly Care Rehabilitation and the Nurse's Role* Brighton, Brighton Healthcare NHS Trust

Sitzia J (1995) 'Volume measurement in lymphoedema treatment: examination of formulae' *European Journal of Cancer Care* 4(1) 11–16

Sitzia J, Dikken C (1996) *NDU Development Proposal 1996–7* Worthing NDU, Day Ward, Worthing Hospital

Smith L (1995) *Long Days Versus Early and Late Shifts: an investigation into the impact of a change in work schedule on performance and well being* Sheffield, Institute of Work Psychology

Stepney NDU (1993) *Video One: Living in Stepney*

Stepney NDU *Annual Report* 1994

Thomas M (1995) *Normal Midwifery for Obstetric House Officers* Royal Bournemouth Hospital Maternity Unit

Truth Ward NDU North Middlesex Hospital 1992–1995

United Kingdom Central Council (1992) *The Scope of Professional Practice* London, UKCC

Vaughan B, Edwards M (1995) *Interface Between Research and Practice* London, King's Fund

Waight S (1992) 'Bedside Handover: breaking down the barriers to effective communication' in Black G *Nursing Developments Work in Progress* London, King's Fund

Wallum R (1995) 'Using care plans to replace the handover' *Nursing Standard* 9(23) 24–26

Walsh D (1995) *Wistow Nursing/Midwifery Development Unit Final Report* Leicester Royal Infirmary NHS Trust

Wandelt M A and Stewart D S (1975) *The Slater Nursing Competencies Rating Scale* New York, Appleton-Century-Croft

Waterworth S (1995) 'Exploring the value of clinical nursing practice: the practitioner's perspective' *Journal of Advanced Nursing* 22(1) 13–17

Waterworth S, Byrne C (1995) 'Benchmarking quality rules' *Nursing Management* 2(3) 13

Watkins S, Theis B (1993) 'Handover needs research' *Nursing Times* 89(35) 12

Worthing NDU *Annual Report* 1993–4

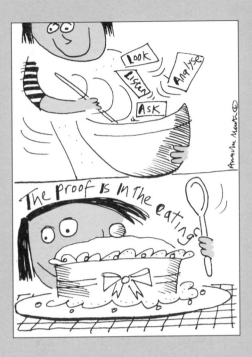

Part 4

PRACTICE-DRIVEN RESEARCH

Nursing research is at an exciting phase in its development having moved from an emphasis on studying nurses in the sixties and seventies to exploring nursing in the eighties and nineties. There is a growing demand for practice to be knowledge based and this shift offers a much needed opportunity to gain insight into the impact of nursing practice on the health and well-being of patients and clients.

Nursing midwifery and health visiting development units are an ideal setting from which to generate clinically driven research. Their quest to ensure that practice is knowledge based not only leads to the use of research in practice, which has been highlighted in section two of this directory, it also opens up the opportunity to refine and explore new ways of working which still need to be tried and tested. One of the most challenging aspects is to generate questions which are directly pertinent in day-to-day work and here NDUs can excel since the more formal research which they have begun to generate has arisen directly from clinical experience.

Skills required to do research well are highly specialised and not always familiar to nurses or colleagues in other health-care disciplines. It is unrealistic to ask practitioners to undertake formal research without ensuring that the requisite skills are at hand so that work is carried out with the rigour that can withstand external scrutiny. Many of the units have formed partnerships with researchers, some of whom have acted as external consultants while others have joined teams and worked alongside them. Both these approaches have advantages and disadvantages which are explored more fully elsewhere (Vaughan and Edwards 1995). In both cases they have played a critical role in helping to shape research questions, refine methods and direct the research. Of equal importance is their role in helping members of the clinical teams gain greater insight into research in order that they can understand the work of others more effectively as well as participate in the process themselves.

Research takes time. While some of the smaller studies have been completed and the findings published, some of the more complex work which was initiated at the outset is only just now coming to an end. The impact of the more formal research from the NDUs has yet to be felt and some of the studies which have been included here are still in progress.

The experiences described in this section have been grouped around work related to exploring the views of service users; studies which seek to clarify the efficacy of new nursing services; studies related to the organisation of care; and a final undefined category. A range of different methods has been employed which encompass both qualitative and quantitative perspectives. While many still view randomised controlled trials (RCTs) as the gold star of research, if the underlying work in identifying relevant concepts and their meanings has not been undertaken then the RCTs are at risk of being undertaken out of context. Thus, many nursing questions lend themselves more readily at this stage to qualitative methods which must take equal place in helping to develop and refine practice.

Focusing on Users

Discovering the views of patients and clients unclouded by the perceptions of health-care workers is critical if services are to be developed which are truly responsive to the needs of those who use them. The work outlined in this section focuses on ways these views have been sought and, while still in the early days of development, these initiatives have already led to changes in practice.

Client and family satisfaction surveys

Worthing NDU has carried out a patient satisfaction survey over an 18 month period, with responses from 175 patients (out of about 200 questionnaires distributed). Patients receiving chemotherapy have not been included as a separate study for this group has been undertaken. The majority of results from both studies have been positive, highlighting issues related to different aspects of care. The latter survey has focused on gaining patients' views on information given (at diagnosis, through treatment and at discharge), facilities, and aspects of medical care and the results will form the basis of future development work. (Sitzia 1993, 1994)

A client satisfaction survey was also undertaken as a management course project by a member of Royal Bournemouth Hospital NDU. One hundred semi-structured interviews were conducted post-natally on an informal basis over a period of 18 months. The women involved had normal deliveries (apart from a small number who had either a Caesarean birth or forceps delivery). Some clients on the high risk unit were included for comparison. The results showed a high degree of client satisfaction while highlighting areas for improvement such as continuity when transition to an obstetric unit is required. It is anticipated that the study will be repeated at intervals to monitor any changes. (Walker *et al.* 1995)

Southampton Children's Outpatient Department NDU has conducted a family satisfaction survey as part of an overall evaluation strategy. Eighteen families were interviewed initially in order to generate subject areas for a questionnaire. This was then distributed to over 400 families, with 243 completed (a response rate of 61%). The questionnaire contained sections on demographic details, information and communication, roles and relationships and rights and empowerment. Feedback from this study was generally favourable with the unit comparing well with other outpatient departments. The evaluation has provided valuable information for planning further strategies to ensure nurses are carrying out the role required by families including introduction of the named nurse scheme to provide continuity and better communication. (see Bartlett and Campbell 1994)

Patient focus groups

As part of Weston Park Hospital NDU's programme to improve the quality of care for patients on the ward, external researchers were commissioned to run a series of independent focus groups with patients. The stimulus for this work was that all the innovations which had been undertaken previously had arisen from concerns of the nurses rather than the patients. The aim of the focus groups was to talk through patients' experiences in an informal context in order to identify areas of satisfaction and potential change. Some of the findings confirmed the views of staff and gave the team confidence with regard to their own perceptions as well as real satisfaction in knowing that work they were doing was valuable. Other points were novel and called for action, such as the plastic on patients' pillows causing sweating and discomfort which has since been dealt with. While it has not yet been possible to respond to all issues raised in the focus groups, (such as the desire of very ill patients to have company and the distress of others at seeing how unwell they are) they have provided a valuable basis from which to plan patient-focused change. The groups are being repeated to see if changes have been well received and also to generate ideas for future work. (see Weston Park NDU Update 1994, Copperman and Morrison 1995)

Children's rights project

Stepney NDU gained an RCN/Gulbenkian award – the Children's Rights in Nursing Award 1994 – to undertake a children's mental health and public health research project. The aim was to identify the main public and environmental health issues for young children aged four to six years living in poverty and deprivation, many of whom do not have English as a first language. It was also an opportunity to explore a methodology for undertaking research with young children. The research was undertaken by the project nurse/clinical leader of the NDU. (see James 1995)

New Nursing Initiatives

With the increasing interest in nursing-led services there is an imperative to explore ways in which these services can be developed to meet need and to assess not only the clinical outcomes but also the acceptability to patients and clients and the cost-effectiveness in both the short and long term. Work is being undertaken in these areas in a range of different settings using a variety of different methods. While it will take some time to gather sufficient data to give definitive answers, early findings are encouraging.

Transfer to the ward from ICU: families' experiences

The point at which families are transferred from ICU is a critical one in their progress, and a study has been undertaken at the Chelsea and Westminster ICU NDU to explore this experience from the families' perspective. The design of the study is based on Parse's emergent research methodology, derived from her Health Becoming theory of nursing (Parse 1981). It takes the form of a phenomenological study (which seeks to explore the meaning of an experience for those involved) describing the experience of having family members transferred to the ward after being in intensive care. The findings are based on the perceptions of four relatives who had been through this process. The common concepts extracted from the participants' propositions were that positive feelings were associated with the transfer which is seen as progress towards health; that past and present experiences can alter the perception of the process; and that good communication and perceived expertise promotes confidence and security but can accentuate feelings of isolation on transfer. The study reveals the complexity of relatives' feelings, and indicates the potential influence that past experience, the actual transfer process and the organisational approach can have on relatives' perceptions of the experience itself. (Mills 1993, 1995)

Single case evaluation, user and GP surveys

As a preliminary to, and as a baseline for, the development of Anticipated Recovery Paths (ARPs) for patients with anorexia, work is being undertaken by Annex NDU on using single case evaluation to describe and illuminate clinical outcomes. Alongside standard outcome measures, individual case studies will be analysed to illuminate certain treatment paths and to provide process evaluation.

In line with its philosophy of user involvement, Annex has commissioned an external consultant to help prepare and carry out a survey of all patients who have used the service since it opened in April 1994. This survey has involved a postal questionnaire, which will be followed by telephone interviews and focus groups. In the longer term it is intended to establish a user forum to play a key role in the evaluation and future development of the service. The result of the survey will be available shortly.

Annex has also surveyed general practitioners whose patients have been treated or assessed in the NDU. A questionnaire was sent out and a response rate of 64% achieved. There was a high level of overall satisfaction with the service, with 75% of GPs rating it as good or excellent. They were also asked about the quality of the information they received and ways in which they would like to see it developed. The key areas identified were direct referral by GPs, emergency assessment and self-referral by patients. These have been offered since mid-April 1996. As a result of the feedback the team are also developing audit targets to make it easier for GPs to identify who to contact for information about patients, to understand the care programme approach and to find out quickly about a patient's disorder, treatment and likely prognosis. (Annex 1996)

Nutrition research

Stepney NDU received an award in 1993 from the Nursing Standard/Dairy Council to undertake a qualitative research project looking at cultural patterns and health beliefs about diet and weaning in Bangladeshi families in Stepney and Wapping and to ascertain health workers' views on weaning advice and health promotion. The project uses focus groups and art activities and is led jointly by a health visitor and a lecturer in primary care. (Buxton 1993)

Stroke and coronary heart disease in South Asian population research

In 1995, Stepney NDU set up a Health Education Authority research programme on stroke and coronary heart disease in the south Asian population. This is a qualitative study to explore cultural health beliefs around the heart and heart disease in the Bangladeshi population in the East End of London. It is anticipated that it will lead to more effective community-based health promotion strategies. This is a joint project between St Bartholomew's Hospital, Princess Alexandra College of Nursing and Midwifery and SNDU, with a dedicated researcher appointed to undertake most of the research. A report is pending from the Health Education Authority. (Stepney NDU Annual Report 1994)

Complementary therapies in nursing

A small-scale research study of the place and practice of complementary therapies in nursing was undertaken by a member of the Oxford 7E NDU. The project was a qualitative case study based on 11 nurses in medical wards. Semi-structured interviews were conducted and analysed using a cognitive mapping technique. Findings indicated that complementary therapies were being widely used but examples of suspect and naïve practice were found. Respondents were unable to provide substantive evidence of the benefits of using such therapies and there was confusion and uncertainty surrounding their safety. The use of aromatherapy was subject to a moratorium following this work; some respondents were concerned about its reintroduction and queried its importance and priority in their workloads. Recommendations from the project included the cessation of complementary therapies until their safe and beneficial use could be ensured; that practice should be based on research, with the need for an empirical basis; and the need for trust guidelines and practice standards. (Oxford Radcliffe Hospital NDU Annual Report 1993–4)

Chemotherapy and side effects

Worthing NDU is conducting a survey by self-report questionnaire on the side effects of drug combinations in chemotherapy treatment to ascertain what patients actually experience when undergoing specific treatment regimes. An internal report on the pilot study is available from the unit which highlights a range of different side effects which patients had not reported verbally. This has already led to changes in the management of side effects for patients. Data collection has been completed for the main study and is currently being analysed. The aim is to use the results of the main study to produce regime specific booklets for the patients.

Although not included as part of this study, patients who received the questionnaire about the side effects also reported a higher degree of feeling 'supported' in response to a wider patient satisfaction survey, which has led the team to consider ways in which this aspect of care could be enhanced.

In addition, factor analysis of the questionnaire has made it possible to refine and simplify the baseline assessment used in the unit making it simpler to use for both patients and staff. (Sitzia *et al.* 1995)

Comparative study of lymphoedema treatments

Worthing NDU is also conducting a trial, using matched pairs, to compare two commonly used lymphoedema treatments (multi-layered bandaging and manual lymphatic draining) in terms of the volume outcomes. These treatments have very different durations, one taking half an hour to complete and the other two hours, and therefore there is a major cost implication as well as an issue of efficacy. Recruitment into the trial will continue until statistical significance is achieved. (Sitzia 1995)

Prevention of stomatitis in patients receiving chemotherapy

In a third proposed study, Worthing NDU is planning research which relates to the use of Sucralfate, commonly prescribed for the treatment of gastro intestinal ulceration, as a prophylactic measure against stomatitis for patients receiving VFU chemotherapy. A double-blind, placebo-controlled, crossover trial is planned as a means of assessing the efficacy of this approach. (Worthing NDU Annual Report 1994)

Survey of water births

The number of water births has been audited in the Royal Bournemouth Hospital NDU over a two-year period. Pool users have accounted for 22% of all deliveries, with nearly 14% having a water birth. Surveys have been carried out by the unit to discover the effects of water on labour and incidence of perineal trauma. While not conducted as randomised controlled trials (RCTs), these studies have indicated that, contrary to published opinion, being submerged in water does not appear to shorten labour and does not reduce perineal trauma. In an ongoing survey, 135 questionnaires are being completed by multiparous women to see how their water births compared to their previous land births, with special focus on post-natal depression and the baby's behaviour. (Royal Bournemouth Hospital NDU Maternity Unit Report 1996)

Psychosocial skills intervention programmes

Tameside and Glossop Mental Health NDU developed a training course in psychosocial intervention techniques based on a problem-centred approach to people with serious mental illness and their families. The training aimed at giving students a broad introduction to the theory that underpins psychosocial interventions and an opportunity to acquire and practise skills under close supervision. (Bagley 1995). The evaluation of this training programme is presently being written up as part of an MSc dissertation.

Evaluation of bridging therapy project

See also page 75

A formal evaluation of the bridging therapy process in the Maudsley NDU has been ongoing. The research has been designed to answer questions about:

- the efficacy of bridging therapy in improving clinical outcomes, particularly in reducing incidence of readmission
- the cost-effectiveness of an extended acute service
- how bridging therapy is seen by clients and primary nurses
- the evaluation of practice and service development
- the process of bridging therapy
- individual and team development

A control group of patients and nurses from elsewhere in the trust has been compared with the experimental group, and the process has been examined by a case study method. This study was delayed when a change in the nature of the client group cared for in the unit led to a higher dependency without an increase in resources. This has not influenced the ethos behind bridging therapy which focuses on early discharge planning, and work is continuing to adjust the process to reflect the change in needs of the client group. It does however highlight the complexity of undertaking clinical research in an environment which is subject to changes beyond the control of those involved in the research. Tentative results from this work have shown an encouraging compliance with medications and lengthening of time between re-admissions. However, these results must be treated with caution until further data are available; this may take some time owing to the organisational changes outlined above.

Noise control project

Ashington (Ward 5) NDU has conducted a study on noise control. This developed from a growing awareness amongst ward staff of the problems posed by noise in hospital, and from a desire to create a more therapeutic ward environment. The NDU's own ward patient satisfaction surveys showed that some patients found noise to be a real problem.

The main findings from the study are: the move to a new hospital appears to have resulted in a reduction of around 15 decibels during the daytime, and ten decibels during the evening and night; there is no significant difference in sound levels when project and comparison wards are compared; at the new hospital, several noise sources continue to cause high sound at various times during the 24-hour period (these include telephones, nurse-call buzzers at bedsides and in toilets, movement of furniture, domestic and cleaning equipment, and kitchen noise).

It was possible to identify three broad groups of patient reaction to noise from the literature review, and to categorise each patient survey accordingly.

Patient Category 1: 'There is no problem with noise'.
Patient Category 2: 'Noise is to be expected in hospital'.
Patient Category 3: 'Noise is a real problem'.

Of the eight patients interviewed, six fell into the first category, one into category two, and one into category three.

The unit is seeking to introduce noise control targeted on the identified sources, and analyse its effectiveness in terms of cost, sound reduction, and patient perceptions. Results should be available in 1997. (see Ashington Annual Report 1992–3)

Fall management study: an action research project

Ashington (Ward 5) NDU has set up a project to identify groups of patients who are at risk from falls, and to investigate possible solutions to the problem. The objectives are:

• to identify risk factors as perceived by nurses, for patients who fall on the project ward, and compare with risk factors identified in the literature

- to evaluate current practice on the project ward, with regard to fall management
- to develop, pilot and evaluate an intervention programme based on existing research and results of the initial study

An action research approach is being used in an attempt to reduce the incidence of falls on the project ward. Data are being collected from a sample of nurses by questionnaire. This will be complemented by semi-focused interviews. Questionnaires and interviews will also elicit patient and family views on fall management so that these can be incorporated into the changes required in the final intervention/ management strategy. (Family perceptions of fall risk have already been identified as being important on the project ward). In the second phase of the study, a strategy will be formulated, implemented and evaluated. This is part of an MSc and a report will be ready in 1997.

Organisation of Care

Another rapidly changing area is the organisation of care and this has formed the basis of research activity within the NDUs. Some of the changes are major ones, such as the introduction of nursing-led in-patient services, while others are focused within the unit themselves, as in the example given of evaluating primary nursing.

Evaluation of the nurse-led in-patient service

A major study is under way on Byron NDU to assess the influence of being cared for in a nursing-led in-patient ward on patient outcomes, using a randomised controlled trial. Patients in the acute wards of the hospital who fit the admission criteria for Byron are randomly allocated to the traditional setting or are transferred to Byron; the purpose and function of the unit are explained and they are offered the choice of the two. Comparisons are then made between the two groups comparing a range of variables that includes length of stay, complications which may be influenced by nursing such as chest and urinary tract infections and skin integrity; degree of independence, degree of well-being, mortality and place of discharge.

Results of the pilot study are very encouraging and show that the patients who are cared for in the nursing-led unit are fairing as well or better on all the variables considered. The full study is now under way and will be completed in 1997. Replication of this work is also being undertaken at the Homerton hospital with a similar evaluation (Alderman 1996). Results of the pilot study on Byron Ward can be found in Griffiths and Evans (1995).

Evaluation of continuity of care in midwifery care

The research aim for Wistow Midwifery NDU has been continuity of care with the theory that 'the establishment of Midwifery Group Practices will lead to increased continuity of midwifery care to women and increased satisfaction for women and midwives.' Consideration was given to the feasibility of employing a randomised controlled trial since it was felt this would appear most credible. However the dynamic nature of the change which was under way made such an approach impossible. A time series design has been employed and a two-pronged approach to the evaluation has been chosen using both quantitative and qualitative data. An economic evaluation has also been attempted but in the absence of any proven mechanism to determine cost it has not progressed.

This work encompasses a comparative study of the different stages in the evolution of change in a before-and-after design involving: a maternal satisfaction questionnaire 36 weeks ante natally and four weeks post natally; obstetric audit outcomes for before-and after-groups; midwifery job satisfaction before and after; measurement of continuity of carer standards.

Maternal satisfaction results indicate women's preference for being attended by a known midwife throughout their care. Similarly, midwives enjoy working in group practices, with more autonomy and opportunity to use their skills to the full. Clinical outcomes indicate similar results to more traditional care approaches.

It also includes an ethnographic interview study of women's experience of care which has provided rich data for future development work focusing on two key themes: namely, seeking ways of ensuring that women feel able to approach staff whom they perceive as being busy and secondly, working further on de-institutionalising the care setting and systems. (Walsh and Atwal 1993–4, Atwal 1996, Walsh 1995)

Evaluation of primary nursing

Bowthorpe NDU has undertaken a study entitled *Primary Nursing from the Patients' Perspective*, to compare primary nursing with another organisational method of care, team nursing. The proposal is to interview a sample of NDU patients after discharge using a relatively unstructured but guided approach. It is hoped to expand the study to involve comparison with patients' views on other wards. The unit is also conducting a study of staff's perspectives on primary nursing. (Bowthorpe NDU Annual Report – year two)

Evaluation of case management

See also page 79

The Royal Victoria Infirmary NDU has been involved in a major research project evaluating the introduction of a case management system and its impact on patient outcomes. This research is being undertaken in conjunction with the University of Newcastle. The evaluation has the following three objectives:

- to describe the processes involved in the introduction of nursing care management and produce a clear operational statement of the requirements for case management
- assess the likely effectiveness of nursing care management for patients and service use
- have a set of tested selection procedures and validated instruments for use in a multi-centre prospective study which will be carried out in the future

The evaluation includes the following aspects:

- a comparison of the pre-implementation and post-implementation patient measures for cohorts of patients
- a measure of anticipated outcomes within the case management project
- a determination of its compatibility with workplace culture
- recommendation of modifications in components, direction and pace of implementation in other areas
- suggestions for priority of managing listed case types

The work is still in an early phase and funds have now been procured from the Medical Research Council (MRC) and the region to continue evaluation over the next two years and early stages of this work are already reported. (Hale 1995)

Survey of skill mix and outcomes of care

The Royal Victoria Infirmary NDU has been part of a national survey undertaken by the health economics unit at the University of York which was concerned with the relationship of skill mix to outcomes of care. The results of this study suggest that there is an improvement in the quality of physical and psychological care when delivered by qualified rather than unqualified staff which has obvious implications when planning the structure of clinical teams. The results have also identified areas for development work within the unit, including the introduction of case management. (RVI NDU Annual Report 1992–3, Car Hill *et al.* 1992).

See also page 79

Outreach primary nursing

Outreach primary nursing research is being carried out by Seacroft (wards V and W) NDU's primary nurses which entails providing follow-up to patients once they have been discharged home. The primary nurses see this as a natural extension of their role to improve discharge procedures and prevent rapid re-admission of some patients. The importance of continuing a therapeutic relationship between the nurse and patient in the person's home has been emphasised throughout this work. A questionnaire is being compiled with the help of a university nurse researcher for semi-structured interviews in the patient's own home. Some problems have been experienced with the progress of this work as some of the nurses involved have moved away, but evaluation of its effectiveness will be an ongoing process. One of the questions considered is the most appropriate time to identify people who would benefit by outreach work. Initially, this was left until the end of the stay in hospital but has now been changed to assessment on admission. (see Gordon 1995)

Organisational mapping

A mapping exercise of the employees of Sheffield City Council has been undertaken with the aim of producing a healthy organisation and reducing work stress. The standard questionnaire SF36 is being used, 2000 of which have been issued to the workforce. The results are being collated by a psychologist. When available, they will be used as a baseline measurement to identify problem areas where occupational health intervention may be required and to enable evaluation of future work. (Rapier 1996)

Developing elderly care rehabilitation and the nurse's role: an action research project

Brighton Homeward NDU has undertook an action research study, the aims of which were to:

- evaluate the work of the ward
- increase the capacity of the nursing team to meet patients' needs so improving the quality of patients' care on the ward
- explore the role of the nurse in the rehabilitation of elderly people, a rapidly developing area of nursing expertise

The action phase was preceded by an interview study of representatives of key groups involved on the ward including patients and carers, nurses and colleagues from other disciplines. Their views were used as a basis for action proposals aimed at developing practice. The process involved facilitated meetings of nurses to discuss the perceptions of patients and carers. Three areas were revealed as in need of urgent attention: information, continuity of care and empowerment of patients. Goals and actions were identified in relation to all three. Following implementation of the action phase over a period of a year, a second group of patients was interviewed. The findings indicated a greatly increased understanding of primary nursing and rehabilitation. In addition, the establishment of the Patients' Forum and other factors had led to a decrease in patients' feelings of vulnerability. However, despite efforts by the nursing team, continuity of care continued to be an area of concern for some patients, particularly night care, and this required further attention.

The project was deemed to have achieved both of its primary aims. First, it increased the capacity of the nursing team to meet patients' needs more effectively and improve the quality of patient care by revealing patients' and carers' perceptions of the ward. Second, although many patients had failed to understand rehabilitation or the rationale behind the unit, subsequent work addressed these shortcomings. In addition, the project showed how effective an action research approach can be in accessing users' views, identifying problems and in bringing about rapid solutions with a consequent improvement in patient care. (see Sheppard 1994, Copperman and Morrison 1995)

Collaborative research links

Chelsea and Westminster ICU NDU was approached by the Director of Nursing Services from the Royal Brompton Hospital with the purpose of developing research links between the two sites. This has resulted in links between the Royal Brompton Hospital and Chelsea and Westminster Hospital Trusts to promote, co-ordinate and develop collaborative nursing research between them. A Nursing Research Link Group has been formed from the Chelsea and Westminster site which includes members from inside and outside the NDU. Collaboration between staff on the two sites has been made a priority. Research activity profiles for both sites have been developed and two directories have been produced: one on sources of funding for nursing research/practice development/post-registration education; and the other on nursing research and development databases. A collaborative research strategy has been developed, the key areas being:

- family/parent/partner/relative satisfaction with care, particularly family-centred care
- nurse-led clinics/services and the nurse's role in health promotion
- patient experiences across interfaces in care provision
- multi-disciplinary team collaborative research opportunities
- nurses' role in the nutritional support of patients
- clinical supervision
- nursing at night
- implications of Integrated Care Pathways (ICPs) for nurses and patients
- how nurses are responding to changing client need within collaborative frameworks
- promoting continence
- the management of inappropriate behaviour

The aim of the strategy is to provide direction for nurses working within the two trusts who may wish to undertake research, and to provide opportunities for both sites to be used for fieldwork. The Nursing Research Link Group meets twice a year, with representation from both sites. Its main role is to act as a resource to members and to maintain an active network through the production of a six-monthly newsletter. (Chelsea and Westminster Intensive Care and NDU Annual Report 1994–5)

Roles

As new services arise so the traditional boundaries of roles will change along with the need to explore different ways of organising work. Critical evaluation of these initiatives in order to gain insight into their efficacy and viability is an important area of study. In this section we have included work which explores nurses' perceptions of new roles, and ways in which their skills can be enhanced alongside an exploration of the introduction of the role of the clinical nurse specialist.

Perceptions and experiences of primary nursing practice

Chelsea and Westminster ICU NDU has completed a study entitled *Nursing Staff's Perceptions and Experiences of Primary Nursing Practice in the Intensive Care Unit (ICU): Four Years On.* Primary nursing has been practised on the unit for four years and during the early stages of implementation an evaluation of staff's perceptions of the system was undertaken. The findings influenced the decision to continue to develop primary nursing which has flourished within the unit. The purpose of this study was to consider how staff perceive primary nursing when well established; what benefits and difficulties for patients, their families, and nurses accrue; and what impact primary nursing has on the nurse's role in ICU. The study design drew on interpretative methodology focusing on staff's perceptions and experiences. A semi-structured questionnaire with open questions was used. All staff were encouraged to participate and a 70% return rate was achieved (n=30). Thematical content analyses were used to analyse the data by generating categories and themes from the data.

The results demonstrated that the majority of the staff felt that the benefits of primary nursing far outweighed the disadvantages. Advantages cited for the patient and the family were: improved rapport, better communication and more in-depth knowledge of the patient and their care. Benefits for the nurse were: increased job satisfaction and sense of achievement, and nurses being able to see things through from admission to discharge. Senior staff felt that another important benefit of practising primary nursing in the ICU setting was a flattening of the hierarchy. Difficulties included: possible greater dependency on the nurse (for the family), and certain negative consequences of caring for long-term patients (for nurses). This supports many of the research findings from other studies in different areas of nursing. (see Manley 1994, Manley *et al.* 1995a, 1995b)

Evaluation of the clinical nurse specialist

A second current research study in the Chelsea and Westminster ICU NDU is entitled: *The Role of the Clinical Nurse Specialist (CNS) in Facilitating the Development of Nurses and Nursing in Providing a Quality Service to Patients: An Action Research Project.* The CNS role has four specific sub-roles (expert practitioner, researcher, educator and consultant), and explicit criteria and competencies are expected including a masters degree/PhD and post-graduate teaching certificate, expert skills and competencies in change management, collaboration, leadership, and facilitation. An evaluation of the role has been conducted using an action research approach which focuses on the emancipatory mode rather than the technical or practical modes (Grundy 1982). Central to this approach is values clarification, reflection and maximum collaboration. A number of action research cycles can be illustrated at various levels: for example, at the macro level an action research cycle can be linked to the unit's general purpose which is in turn represented by the eight objectives the NDU established initially using the process of values clarification.

At an intermediate level, action research cycles link to each of the specific objectives set; for example, the work on developing the unit's quality assurance tools and the development of the staff. Here a number of unstructured interviews have been undertaken with key people who have left the unit for promotion and career progression and a theme arising from these is one of obvious empowerment. At a micro level, research cycles relate to the personal actions of the CNS where staff have formally been collaborating in a review of the clinical nurse specialist's post. Data collection has also included diary keeping by the CNS during the first two years of the project and group discussions on a team by team basis. The emphasis in these discussions has been on what staff found to be helpful or unhelpful, and what they wanted the CNS to do more or less of. Subtle changes in the CNS role have resulted from this. (Manley 1993a, 1993b, 1996)

Reflective practice

A development study on reflective practice within Seacroft (wards V and W) NDU has been formally evaluated by a researcher from the local university. The aim has been to continue to develop nursing staff and their ability to think about nursing practice at a conceptual level, and thus to equip them with the tools to shape and change practice for the better. The group has gone through three phases: reflection on the social reality of nursing (the relationship of the nurse to the organisation); the development of themes emerging from the first phase (focusing on individual client/patient care); and the further refinement of themes. The process is being analysed and will be presented as a research report. In addition, personal development programmes are emerging. The group continues to meet on a fortnightly basis for two hours.

Primary nursing

The West Dorset NDU has undertaken a qualitative study of primary nursing using interviews with nurses on the unit. Findings indicate that it has moved from a functional way of organising care delivery towards re-identifying and restructuring the unique activities of nursing and the central role of caring. Primary nursing has enabled the nurses to identify important nursing skills, knowledge and attitudes towards their work. This has led to the development of a primary nursing course for primary and associate nurses, in partnership with the Institute of Health and Community Studies. The needs of the group are generated through action sets, and the course is spread over a three-month period. The course has now been accredited. (Bournemouth University 1996)

Theoretical Studies

The following studies have explored nursing in a range of different ways in order to gain insight into the nature of the work and throw light on actions which are difficult to explain at first sight. Making explicit the rationale behind such actions, particularly as they relate to direct patient care, remains an important area for study as we continue to develop the service which is offered to patients. Each piece of new work helps to build on this insight.

Perceptions of nursing

A member of Liverpool NDU has undertaken a phenomenological study (after Heidegger) to explore how nurses at different levels of expertise perceive nursing in the 1990s. The study population (12 nurses) was taken from the three wards forming the unit. Six nurses had been qualified for less than a year and six for two or more years. All were asked to keep a reflective diary for six months, and these were used in conjunction with the critical incident technique to help identify and reflect on the positive and negative aspects of nursing. The data were analysed and respondents were then interviewed to validate and expand upon the interpretation. The data highlighted the therapeutic nature of nursing and the value of having qualified nurses at the bedside. It also identified stresses like no time to care and lack of support, and demonstrated a need for all trained nurses to have personal and professional support in the development of their practice. Changes arising from this study have included the introduction of clinical supervision and the way in which primary nursing is employed. (see Boon 1995)

Exploring clinical practice

Liverpool NDU has also conducted 'a preliminary study which has attempted to explore the value of nursing from the viewpoint of practitioners. The objective was to further knowledge and develop insights into nursing practice, identifying concepts central to therapeutic care. Integral to the study was the development of a model for reflective practice' (Waterworth 1995).

Nurses reflected on situations in which they considered they had made a positive difference in a nurse-patient or nurse-relative encounter. The process was assisted by a facilitated two-day workshop on reflective practice, followed by fortnightly seminars.

During the seminars, a member of the nursing team shared a narrative or nursing story about such an encounter. Seminars were taped and transcribed; the sessions were analysed and the analysis validated in subsequent seminars. The analysis has given rise to two broad areas of nursing intervention: supportive/comforting and preventative actions; and to the identification of four dimensions of nursing which can be used to explore the nature of practice more fully, namely: person-centred or focused activities; interpersonal activities; communication and team work. The validation seminars have raised a number of questions, two of which are to be the basis of further research, namely:

- What effect does trying to meet all the patients' individual needs have on the nurse?
- What is the legitimate role of the trained nurse and who legitimises it?

Experience from this study supports the view that more studies are required that empower and transform the participants themselves as they take part in the research process. (Waterworth 1995)

Models of clinical supervision

Tameside and Glossop Mental Health NDU has undertaken a research project exploring models of clinical supervision. Particular emphasis has been given to the difficulty of resourcing clinical supervision, alongside the importance of matching the supervision chosen to the specific needs of different groups. The implementation of initial research recommendations which is sensitive to the needs of the nurses working within the hospital rather than elsewhere within the trust, has taken place and is being further evaluated using a variety of research methods. (Deacon 1994)

Developing a therapeutic milieu

In Brighton CCU NDU work in the first year was directed to the introduction and development of primary nursing, and identified competencies to extend the role of the nurse practitioner in critical care. Two years later links were established with a researcher from the local university and action-oriented research was introduced to illuminate the impact of the therapeutic milieu on different practitioners and relatives of patients cared for on the unit. The findings were reported as case studies, written for, and about, the practitioners. This enabled them to explore areas of their practice which could be enhanced to improve the service they provided. Three areas were examined.

- By fostering an alternative methodological framework, and using a combination of methods, NDU status was used to explore different approaches and take creative and intellectual risks. Video recordings were made of the nurse in action; later she was asked to reflect about her practice to aid the research, but more importantly to help her in her own individual learning. A complex protocol to ensure this work was conducted ethically was developed in conjunction with the multi-disciplinary team on the unit and local ethicists.
- By recruiting staff from the unit as assistants, practitioners were able to develop research and writing skills under the direct supervision of an experienced researcher, yet outside a normal academic environment; research was thus seen to be conducted by nurses in practice rather than by academics in an ivory tower.
- By engaging staff in reflection on their work throughout the data collection process and in the reading of case studies, staff were constantly required to examine what they did and why. In addition, an action learning model was used to discuss emergent issues at every stage. Individual and group review informed the generation and validation of categories, the accuracy and accessibility of material for public review and ensured that the research was conducted democratically. Individual research contracts were held with each participant, and each stage encompassed education, research and development. (Scholes and Moore 1995b)

The impact of the environment on newcomers

The impact of the environment on newcomers was an issue of great debate amongst the practitioners and link teachers to the unit. This case study made clear the concerns of new practitioners and as a result, strategies for the induction of new personnel (medical and nursing) have been fostered and are continuing to develop.

The first stage was to examine how the nurse interacted with the therapeutic milieu of the unit to understand why newcomers and novices were so overwhelmed when they first started work. This clarified working practices which had evolved from experience on the ward, yet defied articulation without attempts to extract meaning. By clarifying procedures, staff found they could explore ways to help junior colleagues gain mastery of their working environment and demonstrate how to make complex judgements. This has been of particular relevance given the national shortfall of experienced critical care nurses, and the recruitment of junior staff to the unit. A full-time education/ development facilitator has been appointed to ensure development continues beyond the life of the original NDU project. A framework for the training of new staff, and accreditation of new skills is in process, which will act as a pathway to the ENB 100 course.

The second stage examined on how the nurse interacted with the patient to illuminate the unique contribution of nursing in critical care. Put simply, because the nurse spent more time with the patient and relatives, he or she developed a very different capacity to 'read' the patient beyond the technological or altered physiological state recognised by other critical care workers. A fundamental distinction between the purpose of the nurse and that of other critical care workers was identified in the third case study: the nurse aimed to maintain a peaceful rested state whilst others concentrated upon pushing the patient to a cured condition, however aggressive the treatments. A further issue which came to light was the way in which doctors and nurses worked: whereas the medical team operated on a system of seeing was believing the nurse functioned more upon feeling was believing (through touch and emotion). These factors further showed how the critical care nurse made professional judgements which drove her caring imperative in her role as patient's advocate. These findings have informed multi-disciplinary debate, particularly in case conferences. (Knight and Scholes 1994)

Making a difference

The aim of this case study was to discover how nurses used self to the advantage of the patient in intensive care. This was the most complex area of practice to disentangle and explore theoretically. It is a part of practice which is understated and undervalued by the nurses themselves and such caring acts are difficult to make explicit. The fundamental concern of the nurse was to bring humanity to the technical nightmare in which the patients found themselves on ITU. Three key categories have become evident namely, humanising the patient, therapeutic presence and therapeutic absence.

From the outset nurses sought both qualitative and quantitative information which was unique to the patient to build a picture which would allow them to personalise care. In coming to know the patient nursing actions and interventions were adjusted in response to an emerging body of knowledge. Gradually (step by step) reactivity was superseded by proactivity and care became less general and more personal, taking into account, for example, personal preferences to touch and familiar sounds and smells. In learning about the person nurses could use this knowledge to help harness the residual senses of the patient and reduce the technical nightmare of ITU.

'Being there' allowed the nurses not only to provide comfort but also to become sensitive to subtle changes in the patient's condition enabling them to either avert a problem or deal with it quickly. While less experienced or less confident nurses (and doctors) would resort to medication for distressed patients, the experts used themselves and their knowledge of the patient to bring calm, using touch talk and personalised actions.

Such actions were so deeply embedded in the nurses' personalities that they were not easily expressed and video recordings were used as a means of illuminating this caring imperative. Using this approach three key elements emerged: first, ways of engaging the patient's attention, second, maintaining that attention and finally, closing the interaction. Touch was used skilfully in these situations and adjusted according to the nurse's knowledge of how tactile patients had been prior to ITU. It was notable that these techniques were observed and replicated by relatives over time while doctors movements were less fluid and more mechanical.

The nurses also used therapeutic absence once they had come to know the patient, judging when to intervene and when to ensure rest. By getting to know patients as human beings with unique likes and dislikes, the nurse develops the confidence to leave them safely unattended whilst still judging correctly when to offer comfort and assistance. The level of knowledge and clinical dexterity used in these circumstances seemed to epitomise excellence in practice : the true art and science of critical care nursing. (Scholes and Moore 1995a)

The case studies demystified many issues surrounding ITU nurses and nursing. For example, ITU nurses signed up to this career pathway because they wanted to be involved in direct, high quality patient care not because they wanted to escape or hide behind technology; nurses attended to equipment but only in order to give more attention to caring aspects of practice; the distinct caring imperative of the critical care nurse frequently put them in a juxtaposition to other critical care workers; critical care nurses had difficulty articulating and valuing the qualitative aspects of the practice which drove their caring imperative. Most importantly, this work demonstrates the continuing social relevance of nursing and the value-added contribution of the nurse above that of a technician. (Knight and Scholes 1994)

Evaluating the NDU through a multi-faceted research approach

Some of the units have a dedicated researcher and a comprehensive programme of research activity to monitor the work of the unit. For example, the programme of work at Glenfield NDU has arisen from their fundamental philosophy which relates to self-care (after Orem 1991). Areas of study have centred around primary nursing, patient education, nurse education, self-medication and the meaning of self-care itself especially the way each aspect can be used to enhance the opportunity for self-care.

primary nursing – This aspect of the research has included: the reformation of primary nursing philosophy; evaluation of nursing roles within primary nursing; evaluation of nurses' perceptions in primary nursing; evaluation of the practice of primary nursing. (see Bell 1993, Furlong 1995, 1996a/b/d)

staff development – This part of the study has entailed an examination of the development and success of a primary nurse development programme using taped reflective discussions between the researcher and course leader as well as a variety of tools to assess changes in the participants' understanding of their role and responsibilities and in the standards of care planning and awareness of personal accountability.

self-care – A working definition of the concept of self-care has been undertaken through a collaborative conference (Furlong 1995, Mason and Furlong 1996) which has led to a base-line for further work involving:

- a phenomenological exploration of the rationale behind adopting the self-care philosophy and the manner in which it is applied in practice. Results suggest that there is still room for patients to take greater control over which aspects of self-care they take responsibility for.
- the examination of patient perceptions of self-care explored through a grounded theory approach. Data are still being analysed but early findings suggest that although patients enjoy self-caring they still look to the nurses for instruction, seeing them as in control.

- nurse perceptions of self-care, illuminated through a phenomenological approach. In this study seven main themes were highlighted, namely involvement, independence, education, encouragement, individualised care, patient role expectation and nurse control. Interesting questions were raised about coercion in self-care on the part of the nurse rather than free choice for the patients.

self-medication – This project evaluates: the cost of self-medication; patient knowledge and compliance; and patient satisfaction as well as nurses' attitudes towards self-medication. A quasi-experimental, longitudinal design compared and contrasted knowledge and compliance with medicine regimes following discharge between patients who had, or had not, self-medicated. There was little difference between these groups and the team speculate that it is the self-care philosophy with its emphasis on patient education which may be the influencing factor. (Furlong 1996)

patient education – The research on patient education involves: the examination of aspects of care including access to information and education from a multi-cultural perspective. This study is in the planning phase.

Changing nursing cultures

Having undertaken many development activities in the first two years of their project, Cartmel NDU was keen to explore the fragile and turbulent culture in which the following developments had occurred: the introduction of clinical supervision, staff appraisal and development plans, quality initiatives, use of information technology and research-based care planning. A literature review on work climates reinforced their belief in the influence such cultures have on work practices.

First intentions were to use a range of methods to explore the views of both the clinical team and others with a vested interest in the unit in order to elicit cultural issues more fully. However it soon became apparent that there was a wealth of work which had already been undertaken which was not fully explicit nor recorded in a way that could be shared more widely. Hence it was agreed instead to document the activities which had already been undertaken by the NDU team all of which have had a significant impact on the ward culture. As a result of this the unit has published a series of six booklets which are available in text and through the Internet, outlining their project work, the steps taken and the impact on their work with guidelines for others. (Gadd 1995, Gadd et al. 1995a 1995b, Gadd and Colgan 1995, Gadd and Mahood 1995a, 1995b)

Unit evaluation project

When the Maudsley NDU was established, the nursing team anticipated undertaking their own evaluation of the unit's project, but the increased workload produced by new service contracts left them with little time to develop the skills needed for designing the research methods or for collection and analysis of data. The review of the research plan resulted in a new approach – a multi-disciplinary study led by nurses which encompasses examining clinical outcomes, using established research tools, exploring nursing practice through repertory grid techniques and analysing the cost of the service with assistance from health economists. This approach made it necessary to recruit additional experts, and a core group evolved to co-ordinate the study. The progress of this study was influenced by organisational changes which led to a major change in the nature of the client group which led to an increase in patient dependency. The processes being assessed had to be adapted to meet the changing needs. This study demonstrates the way in which practice and research must inter-relate in order to be responsive to those changing needs and the flexibility of the team as well as demonstrating how the underlying value of a specific service provision (in this instance bridging therapy) must be adapted to meet local and contextual needs. (Rainsford et al. 1996)

Fostering research

Creating a questioning environment which is conducive to research is part of the ethos of NDUs as demonstrated by the range of work carried out by the ward team of Newcastle NDU, mainly as part of diploma, degree, masters and PhD studies. Areas in which work has been undertaken include:

- discharge planning in the NDU
- the issues associated with the boarding out of patients
- experiencing primary nursing
- the use of nursing models in the NDU
- nurses' perceptions of their work environment

Reports, unpublished dissertations and theses are available directly from the unit for each of these studies which serve to demonstrate how much can be achieved by practitioners who are given the right support and encouragement.

Developing a strategy

Strelley NDU has worked in partnership with an external researcher throughout this project as they have recognised the importance of evaluation of their work from the outset. Recognising the difficulty of assessing outcomes within the field of health visiting they developed an evaluation strategy which has been used as a framework for each initiative. The research co-ordinator has facilitated this process throughout and tools which explore both output (that is changes in practice) and outcomes (that is changes for the clients) have been employed. The team however acknowledge that it has not always been possible to make direct causal relations between the two but it can act as a base line from which further methods of evaluating health visiting can be developed. (Strelley NDU Annual Report 1994, Boyd *et al.* 1995, Brummel and Perkins 1995)

Summary

The complexity of nursing and the knowledge underpinning practice can be seen from the range and breadth of research activity which is described here. In a time when there is a high demand for professional practitioners to be more overt about the rationale on which they base their practice the work which is being undertaken in the NDUs to generate a deeper understanding of nursing and its impact on patients and clients is of vital importance.

However, undertaking research is only part of the picture. Of equal importance is the manner in which the lessons which have been learned are shared with and used by others. There is a critical need for all practitioners to challenge their own practice, question their actions and be prepared to change if information of new and better ways becomes available. Sadly there is still evidence that professional practitioners are slow to change their attitudes and practices (Stocking 1992). This is despite national endeavours to make reliable evidence more readily available through such initiatives as the Cochrane Library and the York Centre for Review and Dissemination and abstracts of reviews of effectiveness, both of whom undertake meta analysis of research in order to collate information for others. Examples of the ways in which NDUs have sought to improve the knowledge base from which they practise were highlighted in section two of this directory. Perhaps the most important feature is an enquiring attitude and a willingness to explore new ways, not for the sake of change but to improve the services which are offered to patients and clients.

The research work which has been undertaken within the NDUs on both a small and large scale, plays a part in the wider picture of seeking greater insight and better ways to contribute to a health service which is sensitive to the needs of users and effective in helping to achieve desired health goals. The challenge is for us to be sensitive and responsive in finding ways to ensure such knowledge is acted on in a thoughtful and effective manner.

References & related reading

Alderman C (1996) 'Taking the Lead' *Nursing Standard* 10(33) 22–23

Annex NDU (1996) *General Practitioner Evaluation* Annex NDU Pathfinder Trust

Ashington Ward 5 NDU *Annual Report 1992–3* Northumberland, Wansbeck District General Hospital

Atwal S (1996) *Internal Report – Ethnographic Design Outcomes* Wistow Midwifery and Nursing NDU, Leicester Royal Infirmary NHS Trust, Leicester

Bagley, I (1995) 'Evaluation of the Tameside Nursing Development Unit for Psychosocial Interventions'. In eds Brooker C and White E *Community Psychiatric Nursing: a research perspective* Chapman and Hall

Bartlett B, Campbell S (1994) *A Family Satisfaction Survey of the Childrens' Outpatient Department* Southampton University Hospitals Trust

Bell G (1993) 'The role of the primary nurse' *Nursing Developments News* 4 p5 London, King's Fund

Boon A (1995) *The Agony and the Ecstasy of Nursing: a summary paper of an unpublished MSc thesis 1994* Royal Liverpool and Broadgreen University NHS Trust

Bournemouth University *Developing Clinical Leadership Course* Bournemouth University

Bowthorpe NDU *Annual Report* Norwich

Boyd M, Marley L, Perkins E (1995) *Poverty and Health Needs: How Can Health Visiting Respond?* Strelley NDU, Nottingham Community Health NHS Trust

Brummell K, Perkins E (1995) *Public Health at Strelley: A Model in Action* Strelley NDU, Nottingham Community Health NHS Trust

Buxton V (1993) 'A healthy start in life' *Nursing Standard* 8(10) 18–20

Car Hill R, Dixon P, Gibb I, Griffiths M, Higgins M, McLaughlin D and Wright K (1992) *Skill Mix and the Effectiveness of Nursing Care* Centre for Health Economics, University of York

Chelsea and Westminster Intensive Care and NDU *Annual Report 1994–5*

Cochrane Database of Systematic Reviews (CDSR) available through CD-ROM

Copperman J, Morrison P (1995) *We Thought We Knew: Involving Patients in Nursing Practice* London, King's Fund

Deacon M (1994) *What Model of Clinical Supervision would be useful for inpatient psychiatric Services?* research monograph no 1. Psychiatric Nursing Research and Development Unit, Manchester Metropolitan University

Dewsbury NDU *Annual Report* 1994

Furlong S (1995) *Self Care Application in Practice* London, King's Fund

Furlong S (1996a) 'An observation of the roles of the primary and associate nurse in practice' *British Journal of Nursing* in press

Furlong S (1996b) 'Primary Nursing: perceptions of what enhances and what diminishes its success in practice' *British Journal of Nursing* in press

Furlong S (1996c) 'Do self-administration of medicines programmes enhance patient knowledge, compliance and satisfaction?' *Journal of Advanced Nursing* 23(6) 1254–62

Furlong S (1996d) 'Practitioners' perceptions of primary nursing' *Professional Nurse* 11(5) 309–11

Gadd D (1995) *Information Technology* Cartmel NDU Mental Health Services of Salford NHS Trust

Gadd D, Colgan L (1995) *Networking: keeping in touch* Cartmel NDU Mental Health Services of Salford NHS Trust

Gadd D, Colgan L, McFadden K, Collins C, Hadcroft D (1995) *Staff Development: Participating in Change* Cartmel NDU Mental Health Services of Salford NHS Trust

Gadd D, Colgan L, McFadden K (1995) *Research Based Care Plans: A Case Study of Research Use by Mental Health Nurses* Cartmel NDU Mental Health Services of Salford NHS Trust

Gadd D, Mahood N (1995) *Clinical Supervision: a time for professional development* Cartmel NDU Mental Health Services of Salford NHS Trust

Gordon A (1995) 'Revolving door system' *Elderly Care* 7(4) 9–12

Griffiths P (1995) 'Approaches to measuring the outcomes of nursing: past, present and future' *Journal of Advanced Nursing* 21(6) 1092–1100

Griffiths P, Evans A (1995) *Evaluating a Nursing-led In-patient Service* London, King's Fund

Grundy S (1982) 'Three modes of action research' *Curriculum Perspectives* 2(3) 23–34

James J (1993) 'Partnerships with Women and Children – partners in health' *Primary Health Care* 3(6)

Knight M, Scholes J (1994) 'The impact of the therapeutic milieu on newcomers and novices to intensive care'. Unpublished report. University of Brighton

Manley K (1994) 'Primary nursing in critical care' in Millar B, Burnard P *Critical Care Nursing: the Care of the Critically Ill* London, Baillière Tindall

Manley K, Welch J, Hanlon M (1995) 'Perceptions of primary nursing by members of the multi-disciplinary team' Chelsea and Westminster Intensive Care and NDU report

Manley K, Hamill J M, Hanlon M (1995) 'Intensive care nurses' perceptions of primary nursing; Four Years On' Chelsea and Westminster Intensive Care and NDU report

Manley K, Cruse S, Keogh S (1995) 'Job satisfaction in intensive care nurses' Chelsea and Westminster Intensive Care and NDU report

Manley K (1996) 'A Conceptual Framework for Advanced Practice : an action research project operationalising an advanced practitioner/consultant nurse role' in press

Manley K (in progress) 'The role of the clinical nurse specialist in the facilitation of nurses and nursing in providing a quality service to patients; Action Research', PhD thesis University of Manchester/Institute of Advanced Nursing Education RCN

Mason S, Furlong S (1996) 'Implementation of an aspect of self care' *Journal of Clinical Nursing* 5(6) 349–352

Mills C (1995) 'Transfer to the ward from ICU: families' experiences' *Nursing in Critical Care* pilot edition 20–24

Mills C (1993) 'The lived experience of families whose family member is transferred from an ITU practising primary nursing to a ward which is not' unpublished dissertation BSc (Hons) in nursing, University of Manchester/Institute of Advanced Nursing RCN

Orem D (1991) *Nursing: Concepts of Practice* (4th ed) New York, MacGraw Hill

Oxford Radcliffe Hospital *Annual Report* 1994–5

Parse R (1981) *Man-Living-Health: A Theory of Nursing* Pennsylvania, John Wiles and Sons

Rapier J (1996) *SF/36/96* Sheffield City Council

Royal Bournemouth Hospital NDU *Maternity Report* 1996

Royal Victoria Infirmary NDU *Annual Report* 1992–3 pp6–8

Scholes J, Moore M (1995a) 'Making a difference: how the nurse uses self directly and indirectly to the patient's therapeutic benefit'. Unpublished report. University of Brighton

Scholes J, Moore M (1995b) 'How the nurse interacts with the therapeutic milieu of the critical care unit'

Sheppard B (1994) *Looking back – Moving Forward; developing elderly care rehabilitation and the nurse's role* Brighton Health Care NHS Trust

Sitzia J (1993) *Patient Satisfaction research project – survey B* pilot study report, Worthing Hospital NDU

Sitzia J (1994) 'Volume Measurement in Lymphoedema Treatment: examination of formulae' *European Journal of Cancer Care* 4(1) 11–16

Sitzia J (1995) 'A study of patients' experiences of the side-effects associated with chemotherapy; a pilot stage report' *International Journal of Nursing Studies* 32(6) 580–600

Stocking B (1992) 'Promoting change in clinical practice in quality in health care' *Quality in Health Care* vol 1, no 1, pp56–60

Strelley NDU *Annual Report* 1994

Walker J M, Hall S M, Thomas M (1995) 'The experience of labour; a perspective from those receiving care in a midwife-led unit' *Midwifery* September

Walsh D, Atwal S (1993–4) *Wistow Nursing Development Unit Report* Leicester

Walsh D (1995) *Wistow Midwifery – Nursing Development Unit Final Report* Leicester

Waterworth S (1995) 'Exploring the value of clinical practice: the practitioner's perspective' *Journal of Advanced Nursing* 22(1)13–17

Weston Park Hospital NDU *Update* 1994

York Database of Abstracts of Reviews of Effectiveness available through CD-ROM

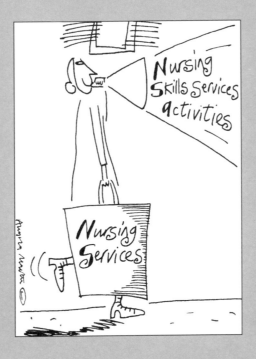

Part 5

DISSEMINATION AND MARKETING

An important facet of the endeavours of all the NDUs has been to disseminate their good practice, both within the trusts and organisations where they are located, and on a national and in some cases international basis. The services of the NDUs are clearly not only for the benefit of the local patients and clients, and sharing their experiences both formally and informally has been an important aspect of their work. The ethos of NDUs is the testing of innovations, the utilisation of research and learning what works in the best interests of patient care. The experiences of the units can be of great value to other service users and providers. They are making knowledge about their good practices known and more widely available and many of them have developed extensive strategies for publicising what they are doing and how they are achieving their goals, as well as the positive and negative lessons learnt in the process.

Some units keep records of the range and type of contact they have both within and external to their own trust which has formed the basis of central evaluation of this aspect of the work. Such records are difficult to maintain and probably do not capture the full range of activity but, early analysis indicates that they are very active not only in the more formal aspects of dissemination but also in responding to phone calls, visits, enquiries and requests for advice about particular aspects of their work (Payne 1996).

Shared work has also taken place between the units. For example, the team on Anston Ward at Rampton have sought advice from the Annex NDU to gain skills in supporting people with eating disorders. Some cohorts of NDUs have formed their own geographically-based support groups in order to share experiences and provide an opportunity for shared problem solving. Help has also been sought from many of the units in supporting other people who are interested in developing their own NDUs and in some instances informal peer review has been undertaken within this area.

One important aspect which appears to have arisen as a result of the programme as a whole is an increasing awareness of the way in which nursing midwifery and health visiting development units can act as a trigger for the development of services which are offered to patients. This growing interest can be demonstrated by, the popularity of the publications which have appeared and in particular the high interest in the open learning pack *Nursing Midwifery and Health Visiting Development Units – a guide* (Freeman 1996) which has been developed as a means of sharing the experiences of the NDUs. In the same way the interest in NDUs which is reflected in enquiries to the Nursing Development Network shows a continuing awareness of this approach to practice development.

Dissemination and marketing can be viewed along a continuum, at a micro level within the unit itself and the local trust and at a macro level where both the specific project work and the concept of NDUs has raised a high degree of interest nationally and internationally.

Strategies for Dissemination and Marketing

At the outset of this programme workshops were offered to the NDUs to help them to devise an overall strategy for dissemination and marketing, pulling out the key messages to share, the target audiences with differing interests and the techniques they could use. As a result, many of the units developed specific plans, an example of which is given below alongside further examples of the different communication processes used at such as seminars and conferences; documentation and publications; media and technology and external links and relationships.

Communication strategy

In the early days of working as an NDU the Glenfield team developed a strategy for communication within and beyond the unit with the following objectives:

- To ensure that all nursing staff working in the unit understand: (a) what an NDU is; (b) what research/projects the NDU is going to be involved in; (c) what their role/responsibilities are within the unit
- To ensure that our patients: (a) know that we are an NDU and what the work of the unit involves; (b) will feel able to participate if they desire to in, for example, the research activities
- To facilitate understanding within the multi-disciplinary team of what an NDU is and the research and practice developments involved
- To stimulate interest in and understanding about the work of the NDU across the cardiology unit
- To stimulate interest in and understanding about the work of the NDU across the trust
- To inform and create interest within practice areas in the local hospitals about the existence and work of the NDU
- To inform and create interest across the purchasers (e.g. GPs and health authorities), referrers (e.g. other hospitals) and colleges of nursing etc. about the existence and work of the NDU
- To facilitate recognition as an NDU nationally

Actions to meet the objectives were specified as well as time scales within which or by which the action would take place. Evaluation was also built in and their success can be seen in the range of publications, visits and interest in their work alongside continuing support from their trust on completion of the external funding. (Communication Strategy – Glenfield NDU Leicester)

Multiple dissemination strategies

Typical of many of the units, Royal Bournemouth Hospital NDU has used a variety of approaches to disseminate activities such as: participation in conferences as speakers; articles in journals; hosting visits; information packages for other professionals; choices leaflet for clients; annual presentations at quality assurance conferences within the trust; visits to local general practitioners to increase their awareness of the work of the unit, as well as the development of a learning pack to assist other service providers to plan changes to their maternity services. Their final report of the project, which is available from the unit, has summarised both the development work and many of these activities. (Royal Bournemouth Hospital NDU Annual Report 1996)

Marketing group

See also page 5

Chelsea and Westminster ICU NDU established a marketing group to generate and co-ordinate marketing strategies, and to market the unit internally via the multi-disciplinary team, the trust and the stakeholders, and externally on a national and international basis. Strategies for marketing and dissemination include an introduction pack for new members; involvement of unit staff as consultants in trust projects; the link nurse programme to improve unit and trust communications; monthly primary nurse open afternoons and an annual conference. (Chelsea and Westminster Intensive Care and NDU Annual Report 1994–5)

Seminars, Conferences and Workshops

Seminars and workshops are a common feature of the majority of NDUs and many have also organised conferences as a means of sharing their experiences with others. Skills have been gained through these processes, not only in the management of such events but also in the presentation of material to people from a range of different backgrounds. Some examples of these activities are given below.

Seminar programme

A common approach to dissemination is that of seminars and Ashington (Ward 5) NDU uses such a programme to this end. Their aim is to provide an opportunity for nurses and other professional carers or therapists to get together and learn about new approaches in order to encourage the spread of best practice in the light of the latest research. The initial seminars have been attended by nurses from hospital and community services including nursing and residential homes. This has been a very positive development, providing a forum for exchange of ideas and contributing to mutual understanding of the services provided. This meeting of front-line clinical staff from the different provider agencies is a step in the direction of a truly seamless service with shared learning. The seminar programme provides a good quality, low-cost method of building up the required evidence of professional development in fulfilment of the UKCC PREP requirements. Most seminars are led by staff from the NDU who have developed specialist knowledge or expertise in the subject area. (see Ashington Annual Report 1992–3)

Conferences

The number of conferences which have been organised by the NDUs is too great to list individually but brief descriptions beow show the wide area of activity.

Wistow Midwifery NDU has held a national conference for midwives which was so heavily subscribed that it was repeated a month later. The conference focused not only on the research findings but also gave a pragmatic and honest report of the complex changes required at an organisational level on such issues as the needs of part-time staff, and midwives who do not drive, while still aiming to meet national targets for continuity of care. In addition, the project leader responded to over 20 invitations to speak at various maternity units throughout the UK over the final six months of the project.

Anston Ward NDU has also been working with and responding to both the trust initiatives and the staff education centre. A major conference focusing on women in forensic care attracted a wide audience from a range of different backgrounds including commissioners; this was particularly relevant as the change in management of forensic services approaches.

Chelsea and Westminster NDU have held conferences annually to share their experience in intensive care as well as developments in their more formal research work. These events have all been well attended and much of the work of the unit in, for example, introducing primary nursing to an environment which has a quick throughput of patients who require highly complex technical care has been drawn on by other units in their own developments.

Seacroft (V and W wards) NDU held a very successful conference for nurses working in mental health, again drawing on their specialist expertise in this area as it relates to practices such as reminiscence and personal development using reflection in, and on, action. (Graham 1995) They also raised considerable debate at this event about the advantages and disadvantages of generic and specialist practice which is currently of wide professional interest.

Workshops and study days

Workshops and study days have also been held by many of the NDUs which have enabled units to accommodate the large number of enquiries they receive. For example, Byron ward runs regular pre-planned seminars to offer people who enquire into the nursing-led services rather than responding in an ad hoc way to each request which is disruptive to the day-to-day running of the unit.

Other examples of workshop activities include:

- *West Dorset NDU* has run regular workshops on primary nursing, clinical supervision, stress management, complementary therapies and therapeutic touch for participants within and outside the unit; thus the work which has been developed within the unit has been made accessible to a much wider audience. (West Dorset NDU Annual Report 1995)

- *Worthing NDU* has also organised local study days on specialist subjects. For example, they have held a number of oncology days for local nurses, which have proved very popular and informative. This work is ongoing and helps to ensure that the skills they have developed in the day-care services can also be made available to patients receiving care elsewhere. (Worthing NDU Annual Report 1994–5)
- *Liverpool NDU* has established, among others, a series of workshops on clinical supervision, and this programme has now been taken over by the Phoenix Unit, the trust's training and development department. This demonstrates one way in which the NDU has acted as a pilot to develop a specific area of work which has then be taken up on a wider basis in order that others can benefit. (Royal Liverpool and Broadgreen University Trust NDU 1995)

See also page 150

Road shows

As an interesting variant, and as part of Cartmel NDU's networking strategy, two road shows were held, one at the Children's Hospital and the other within their own trust, to disseminate work being carried out on the unit. The road shows, which were run and organised by the NDU team, were widely advertised via invitations to clinical managers and wards and by the use of flyers. Various information about the unit was displayed and staff were on hand to facilitate visitors understanding of the nature, philosophy and aims of the NDU and to provide details about each of the project areas. At each venue the idea was to create an informal and relaxed atmosphere in order to promote sharing of good practice. The road shows were evaluated by the use of a short questionnaire with positive results, indicating that many participants found them informative and had learnt things they felt could be put into practice in their own setting. (Gadd and Colgan 1995)

Documentation and Publications

The skills required for writing reports for publications or even care plans are challenging for many nurses. They are more familiar with sharing their views and ideas verbally rather than committing them to paper and the development of writing skills has been an area of personal development for some of the NDU teams. However as the ideas presented below demonstrate, many units have developed excellent skills in written communication.

Reports plans and publications

A range of documentation has been used to make the work of units more visible. For example, the annual report and its accompanying executive summary is used by Wistow Midwifery NDU as a marketing tool and is sent to selected target groups. Summary reports of their work are available directly from the unit. (Walsh 1995)

Stepney NDU have used their interim project report as a means of providing information to a wide range of people with an interest in their work. It has been circulated both within and outside the unit and resulted in much widespread interest. (Stepney NDU Annual Report 1994)

Seacroft (wards V and W) NDU and Homefield Place NDU, amongst others, both have a quarterly newsletter, mainly for local dissemination. In the case of Seacroft this is also sent to a list of contacts on their database.

Publication in journals is obviously another way of disseminating work and achievements. Seacroft (wards V and W) NDU was very active in this area and agreed a commission with the journal *Elderly Care* to write a series of articles about their work. They have also recognised the importance of business plans as a way of both disseminating their activities and showing how the unit is seeking to be part of a market. (Seacroft (wards V and W) Second Annual Report 1994)

As well as the range of internal documents many of the units have published their work either in the nursing press or elsewhere. Many, including Homeward, Strelley and Glenfield have registered publications which can be purchased directly from the unit. Cartmel has opened a page on the Internet and also provide hard copy. Other units have published in the nursing press or been the subject of feature articles themselves.

A novel publication has been the production of the *Living in Stepney* video which was a major piece of work for the Stepney NDU during 1993. The positive response to this film suggests that audio-visual information is effective and popular with local people. It also provides an accessible means of communication for those whose first language is not English.

Publications have been mentioned throughout this text and are given in full in the reference list. Over the past four years a very large number of reports, features and articles which have arisen from the work of the units have been published in both specialist and general journals. However, some of the reports from the longer research projects are only just coming to fruition and there will be a growing number of publications in the coming year.

Media and Technology

To ensure that new developments are shared with the general public as well as other health-care professionals press releases have been issued and journalists invited to some of the initiatives. This is a relatively new approach for most nurses but offers an excellent opportunity to share their expertise with a wider audience and help the public gain insight into the way in which they work.

Media

The media have been used in many instances as a means for dissemination. For example, Byron NDU achieved publicity for the unit through high coverage in nursing (*Nursing Times, Nursing Standard*), medical (*BMJ* and *GP* magazines) and national press (*Observer, Guardian, Daily Mail*). However, the most extensive coverage followed publication of *Evaluating a Nursing-Led Inpatient Service* (Griffiths and Evans 1995) with reports on BBC Breakfast News, BBC Newsroom South East, Carlton, BBC Radios 2, 4 and 5, Independent Radio News, Classic FM, GLR and local radio stations. Extensive coverage in the local press has been particularly valuable in making the service known locally to both health-care workers and potential patients.

Worthing NDU featured prominently in the Channel Four programme *Pulse* which explored the expanding role of nurses within the NHS. While it was both time-consuming and challenging for the team to become involved in work of this nature it was very successful in bringing the developing contribution which nurses are making in health-care to the attention of the public.

Locally, many of the units have received press coverage. Bowthorpe NDU gained publicity for its activities on local news and in the local press and the midwifery unit at Bournemouth has received wide coverage in local papers and featured in regional television documentaries.

There has been a tendency for nurses to restrict dissemination of their work to nursing audiences rather than through multidisciplinary routes, to management forums and the wider public. The importance of sharing widely cannot be underestimated, especially within the current market-driven NHS, and some of the examples outlined above demonstrate ways in which this can be achieved.

External Links and Relationships

Finally, units illustrate an array of different activities which are geared towards the establishment and promotion of external links and relationships. Some of the units have an overall strategy for networking as shown in the first example.

Networking

Cartmel NDU developed a networking strategy on three levels – local, regional and national. However, it was realised that the survival of the unit would depend on the ability to network locally within the trust rather than on a national level so the project manager from the Centre for Practice Development within the trust was asked to chair the networking group. Nurses from a range of clinical specialities joined the group to examine networking possibilities with other nurses in their own clinical area and a link person within each area was appointed. Apart from this, secondment of staff to the unit has been both popular and productive. On a regional and national level, visitors were received and requests for information met.

Three members of staff have been invited to join steering groups of other Nursing Development Units and specific requests for consultancy visits have been made. The national conference which Cartmel NDU held has also been responsible for establishing networking between NDUs using the Internet. It is to Cartmel's credit that the unit has now been closed and the client group for whom they cared re-housed, which was a fundamental aim from the outset. However, interest in NDUs remains high in the trust and it is anticipated that work of this nature will continue in the future. (Gadd and Colgan 1995)

Open days and going out to the people

Many NDUs encourage people to come to the units to find out about their work whilst members of the team visit other sites in response to requests. Truth Ward NDU has held open days aimed at disseminating work internally and externally and good support has come from nurses externally and from the multi-disciplinary team. However one difficulty common to many units has been gaining the interest of nursing colleagues locally, following the adage 'you cannot be a prophet in your own town'. This may be due to a perceived elitism or the misconception that NDUs have additional resources and are treated in a different way from other units. Many strategies have been used to overcome this such as personal visits to colleagues to share ideas and information, offering and seeking help and involvement, distribution of local news-sheets and information leaflets. (Truth Ward NDU 1992–5)

Dewsbury NDU have a planned programme of visits to the A and E department for schoolchildren, cubs, scouts and others. This offers them the chance to see how the department works and what the equipment looks like. Many children follow up projects at school which is one way of helping the general public gain insight not only into the work of nurses but also the type of services which are available in an accident and emergency department.

In addition, Dewsbury ran a health bus visiting town centres and car-boot sales with nurses demonstrating skills and teaching health and safety awareness. Market stalls have been run in the town centre to increase awareness of asthma in the community. First aid and safety courses are offered at the local sports centre to the over 50s. Funding is no longer available for the bus but plans are under way to continue health promotion activities at local supermarkets, shopping entrance areas and elsewhere. (Dewsbury NDU 1995)

Outreach work and consultancy

Worthing NDU has been involved in outreach work and the facilities and resources of the NDU have been used by many other units in the trust. A researcher has been part of the team over the past three years and his skills in data analysis and service evaluation have been called on widely. It is anticipated that this service will soon be actively promoted although the researcher's home base will remain within the NDU. (Worthing NDU Annual Report 1994–5)

Following extensive publicity Byron NDU has received many requests for further information. In particular the team has been invited to act as consultants to another unit wishing to establish a similar nurse-led service who are now replicating both the implementation and the research following the model learned from the Byron experience. (see Griffiths and Evans 1995, Alderman 1996)

East Berkshire NDU has experience of providing consultancy to learning disabilities nurses. In particular they have responded to requests from another trust for the accreditation of two of their homes on the basis of NDU criteria. This resulted in the preparation of a joint article for publication with the other trust. (Balkizas *et al.* 1995)

Working with charities and self-help organisations

Annex NDU has used its connections with the Eating Disorders Association (a national charity) to develop and disseminate its work. Information about Annex has been regularly included in the EDA newsletter and information about the NDU is given out on the charity's help line. Team members have also given talks to self-help groups.

Many of the patients in Annex NDU are seen as extra contractual referrals which makes marketing a part of their day-to-day work. An information booklet about the service is available, as are information leaflets for the patients. Information has been prepared for other nurses who are interested in this type of work and a quarterly newsletter is sent out internally and externally. (Jowett 1996)

Similarly, the work undertaken in Michael Flanagan NDU led to the development of a free-standing service in the trust, SCOPE, which provides care for people who were subject to abuse in the past. (Holly 1996)

Contribution to trust developments

In common with many of the NDUs, Truth Ward NDU has linked with the work of the trust in a number of ways: in looking at clinical supervision, the named nurse initiative, documentation, setting up of stroke and cardiac rehabilitation programmes and being involved in disseminating good practice based on research. They have also contributed to trust programmes for expanding nursing competence in advanced nursing skills such as IV cannulation, venepuncture, confirmation of expected death and limited prescribing. (Truth Ward NDU Report 1992–5)

Staff of Weston Park Hospital NDU have been active participants in the trust's development groups, with the NDU taking the lead on many trust-wide initiatives. They contributed to the setting up of a regional peripheral blood-stem cell harvesting service. (Weston Park Hospital NDU Brochure)

Ward project leaders in West Dorset NDU have been involved in trust committees such as wound management, care standards groups, infection control, nursing strategy and clinical directorate meetings.

Following issues which arose from focus group work Weston Park NDU has submitted a proposal to instigate a young persons' unit as an extension of their own ward. This proposal has been presented to the trust board, the hospital cancer care appeal and the Teenage Cancer Trust. Plans to implement the proposal are under way.

Collaboration

Collaboration is the essence of the external relationships. This has been on a local community basis, with other units, and sometimes even internationally.

For example, Strelley NDU (Health Visiting) has undertaken a collaborative project with a local supermarket in order to raise awareness of the issues surrounding a balanced diet, matching nutritional needs with affordable products. A *Healthy Eating on a Budget* day was organised by a multi-agency, multi-disciplinary group in which commercial and voluntary sectors joined the statutory sector. Simple cheap recipes were produced using pictorial aids and tastings and low-cost menus were available. The supermarket had an estimated 3000 customers that day and there was also coverage in the local newspapers. This programme led to a community breakfast initiative in a local school in collaboration with dieticians and colleagues working in health promotion. (Strelley NDU Annual Report 1994)

Four local NDUs – Brighton Homeward, Worthing, Brighton CC and Seaford – have linked to provide support for the clinical leaders, but the success of a workshop run jointly for all members of the four NDUs will hopefully lead to other events for all nurses. The workshop was chaired by a project officer from the King's Fund, and focused on integrating newer nurses to the NDUs and finding out their views on research-based care and development opportunities in NDUs.

Newcastle NDU has been collaborating with Karen Zander (Principle of Case Management in Boston, USA) to introduce case management into the United Kingdom. The unit is now a member of the international expert user group. (Royal Victoria Infirmary NDU 1993–4)

Another example of collaboration is the several planned education programmes supported by the Liverpool NDU that are run in conjunction with Phoenix Development (the training and development department of the trust), and include:

- clinical leadership and clinical supervision programmes (Waterworth, 1995b)
- supportive therapies education, ENB N17 accredited course
- HIV awareness training
- clinical competence workshops

These both emanate from and support the work of the NDU. (Royal Liverpool and Broadgreen University trust NDU 1995)

SUMMARY

Dissemination of information and marketing is an issue which is unfamiliar to many health-care workers who feel it is neither pertinent nor appropriate to their day-to-day practice. Yet if we, as nurses, do not share information with professional colleagues and service-users then we will limit effective collaboration and the extent to which we can ensure that nursing skills are used to their greatest extent. Clinical leaders of the NDUs have come to the conclusion that this area of work was, or should be, everyone's business and some of their experiences are drawn together in a publication related to the work of the units. (Jowett 1996)

Some people have said that it is difficult for nurses to share their work because we do not have a common language to describe what we do (Lawler 1991) but from the examples given here it is evident that, given the confidence and the skills nurses can, and do, work very effectively in this area. It is through endeavours such as these that a steady increase in the number of new nurse-led services is now reaching patients, bringing together all that is good in nursing and encompassing a wider range of skills.

One of the key characteristics of NDUs has been the dynamic way in which they respond to demands and challenges, seeing change as a way of life and being prepared to develop the services they offer in response to patients' needs. Yet recent surveys (DoH 1993, Bryant 1993) still suggest that of the many innovative areas of practice development made by nurses, few have been brought to the attention of purchasers or commissioners. Service contracts are now part of the NHS culture and as this system becomes more sophisticated the importance of ensuring that the nursing contribution is clearly laid out becomes more and more important. Talking about what we do, being proud of our achievements while still recognising our limitations, finding ways of linking the impact of our care to the outcome for patients and helping people understand the meaning of what nurses do does, indeed, become everyone's business.

References & related reading

Alderman C (1996) 'Taking the Lead' *Nursing Standard* 10(33) 22–23

Ashington NDU Ward 5 *Annual Report* 1992–3, Wansbeck District General Hospital

Balkizas D, Morton S, and Holdgate M. (1995) 'Peer accreditation of a development unit' *Nursing Standard* Vol 9 no 28 25–27

Bryant J (1993) *The Professional Nursing Contribution to Purchasing; a Study by the King's Fund College* Leeds National Health Service Management Executive

Chelsea and Westminster Intensive Care and NDU *Annual Report* 1994–5

Department of Health (1993) *Targeting Practice – the Contribution of Nurses, Midwives and Health Visitors* London Department of Health

Freeman R (1996) *How to become an NDU* London, King's Fund

Gadd D, Colgan L (1995) *Networking: keeping in touch* Cartmel NDU, Mental Health Services of Salford NHS Trust

Glenfield NDU Leicester *Communication Strategy*

Graham I (1995) 'Reflective Practice: Using the Action Learning Group Mechanism'. *Nurse Education Today* 15(1) 28–32

Griffiths P, Evans A (1995) *Evaluating a Nursing-led In-patient Service* London, King's Fund

Holly C (1996) 'Focus on Need' *Nursing Times* 92(3) 46–47

Jowett S (1996) *Every Nurse's Business: the role of marketing in service delivery* London, King's Fund

Lawler J (1991) *Behind the Screens* Melbourne, Churchill Livingstone

Royal Bournemouth Hospital NDU *Maternity Unit Report* 1996

Royal Liverpool and Broadgreen University Trust NDU (1995) *Final Report*

Royal Victoria Infirmary NDU (1993–4) *Annual Report*

Seacroft (wards V and W) *Second Annual Report* (1994)

Stepney Nursing Development Unit *Annual Report* 1994

Strelley NDU (1994) *Changing Needs, Changing Minds, Changing Practice: Annual Report* Nottingham

Truth Ward NDU North Middlesex Hospital *Report* 1992–5

Walsh D (1995) Wistow Midwifery/ Nursing Development Unit *Final Report*

Waterworth S (1995) *Clinical Supervision: Developing a Model (part one)* Royal Liverpool and Broadgreen University Trust

West Dorset NDU (1995) *Annual Report*

Weston Park Hospital NDU brochure, Sheffield

Worthing NDU *Annual Report* 1994–5

Appendix: Nursing, Midwifery and Health Visiting Development Units

The names and addresses of the NDUs whose work has contributed to the development of this directory are given below. However, it should be noted that, as time has moved on, trust amalgamations have occurred and service contracts have altered, so not all units are still functioning in this way. Furthermore, as the interest in NDUs continues to grow, there is an increasing number of new units emerging, some of which can be identified through the Practice and Research Development Network of the King's Fund. Should you wish to make contact with a NDU with similar interests to you and are experiencing difficulty in finding the appropriate address, please do ring the Network Administrator on 0171 307 2668 in order that we can search the current database for relevant information.

COMMUNITY UNITS

Andover NDU

Community nursing – district nursing and community hospital services

Charlton Road Health Centre
Charlton Road
Andover
Hampshire
SP10 3LD

Tel: 01264 358 811

Stepney NDU

Community nursing – district nurses/ health visitors

Steels Lane Health Centre
384 Commercial Road
London
E1 0LR

Tel: 0171 790 7171

Strelley NDU

Health visiting

Strelley Health Centre
c/o Linden House
261 Beechdale Road
Aspley
Nottingham NG8 3EY

Tel: 01602 296 911

MENTAL HEALTH UNITS

Annex NDU

Mental health and anorexia nervosa

Harewood House
Springfield Hospital
61 Glenburnie Road
London
SW17 7DJ

Tel: 0181 682 6338

Anston NDU

Forensic psychiatric care

Anston Ward
Rampton Hospital
Woodbeck
Retford
DN22 0PD

Tel: 01777 248 321

Cartmel NDU

Mental health – long-term care

Mental Health Services of Salford
Bury New Road
Prestwich
Manchester
M25 7BL

Tel: 0161 773 9121

Homefield Place NDU

Mental health and older people

Homefield Place
Homefield Road
Seaford
East Sussex
BN25 3DG

Tel: 01323 490 770

Maudsley (ES3) NDU

Mental health acute

Eillen Skellern 3
Maudsley Hospital
Denmark Hill
London
SE5 8BX

Tel: 0171 703 6333

Michael Flanagan NDU

Mental health and addiction – day care services

Mental Health Foundation
St George's Hospital
Corporation Street
Stafford
ST16 3AG

Tel: 01785 57888

Seacroft (Wards V & W) NDU

Mental health and older people

Seacroft Hospital
York Road
Leeds
LS14 6UH

Tel: 0113 280 3372

Tameside & Glossop Mental Health NDU

Mental health acute

Psychiatric Day Hospital
Community & Priority Services
NHS Trust
Tameside General Hospital
Fountain Street
Ashton-upon-Lyne
OL6 4EW

Tel: 0161 331 5097

LEARNING DISABILITY

East Berkshire NHS Trust NDU

Learning disabilities – behavioural problems

Behavioural Support Team
Church Hill House
Bracknell
Berkshire
RG12 7EP

Tel: 01344 422 722

Witney (Learning Disabilities) NDU

Learning disabilities

Post Office Chambers
Market Square
Witney
Oxon
OX8 7LN

Tel: 01993 774 045

MIDWIFERY UNITS

Royal Bournemouth Hospital NDU

Midwifery led services

Maternity Unit
Royal Bournemouth Hospital
Castle Lane East
Bournemouth
BH7 7DW

Tel: 01202 303626

Wistow Team (LRI) NDU

Midwifery integrated services

Leicester Royal Infirmary
Maternity Hospital
Infirmary Square
Leicester
LE1 5WW

Tel: 0116 254 1414

GENERAL UNITS – ACUTE CARE

Ashington (Ward 5) NDU

General medicine

Wansbeck District General Hospital
Woodhorn Lane
Ashington
Northumberland
NE63 9JJ

Tel: 01670 521212

Bowthorpe NDU

Acute medicine for the elderly

Bowthorpe Ward
West Norwich Hospital
Bowthorpe Road
Norwich
NR2 3TU

Tel: 01603 288 493

Glenfield (Ward 33/CCU) NDU

Cardiology

Ward 33/CCU
Cardiology Department
Glenfield Hospital
Groby Road
Leicester
LE3 9QP

Tel: 0116 2871 471

John Radcliffe Hospital NDU

General medicine/nursing

Ward 7E
John Radcliffe Hospital
Headley Way
Headington
Oxford
OX3 9DU

Tel: 01865 220 894

Royal Victoria Infirmary NDU

Orthopaedic trauma and rehabilitation

Orthopaedic Unit
Ward 22
Newcastle General Hospital
Westgate Road
Newcastle upon Tyne
NE4 6BE

Tel: 0191 273 881

Truth Ward NDU

Acute medical care

North Middlesex Hospital
Sterling Way
Edmonton
London
N18 1QX

Tel: 0181 887 2750

West Dorset NDU

Acute medical care

Maud Alexander Ward
Weymouth and District Hospital
Weymouth
Dorset DT4 7TB

Tel: 01305 760 022

GENERAL UNITS – NON-ACUTE CARE

Byron Ward NDU

Nursing-led service

King's Healthcare (Dulwich site)
East Dulwich Grove
London
SE22 8PT

Tel: 0171 346 6166/6169

Homeward Rehabilitation NDU

Rehabilitation of elderly patients

Brighton General Hospital
Elm Grove
Brighton
East Sussex
BN2 3EW

Tel: 01273 696 955

Southport NDU

Care of the elder/rehabilitation

Southport General Infirmary
Paton Ward
Scarisbrick New Road
Southport
PR8 6PH

Tel: 01704 547 471

GENERAL UNITS – SPECIALIST CARE

Brighton Critical Care NDU

ICU/CCU

Royal Sussex County Hospital
Level 7
Eastern Road
Brighton
BN2 5BE

Tel: 01273 696 955

Chelsea & Westminster NDU

Intensive therapy unit

Chelsea & Westminster Hospital
Fulham Road
London
SW10 9TH

Tel: 0181 746 8516/8

Day Ward Worthing Hospital NDU

Oncology day care

Day Ward
Worthing Hospital
Park Avenue
Worthing
West Sussex
BN11 2DH

Tel: 01903 205 111

Dewsbury Accident & Emergency NDU

Accident & Emergency

Dewsbury and District Hospital
Healds Road
Dewsbury
West Yorkshire
WF13 4HS

Tel: 01924 465 105

Liverpool NDU

Haematology/surgery

7Z Link
Royal Liverpool University Hospital
Prescot Street
Liverpool
L7 8XP

Tel: 0151 706 2231

Southampton NDU

Paediatrics out-patients

Children's Out-Patients' Department
Southampton General Hospital
Tremona Road
Southampton
SO9 4XY

Tel: 01703 794 469

Weston Park NDU

Oncology

Ward 3
Weston Park NHS Trust
Whitham Road
Sheffield
S10 2SJ

Tel: 0114 2670 222

OCCUPATIONAL HEALTH UNITS

Sheffield Occupational Health NDU

Occupational health

Sheffield City Council
Town Hall
Pinstone Street
Sheffield
S1 2HH

Tel: 0114 273 4097